STAYING FIT OVER FIFTY

CONDITIONING FOR OUTDOOR ACTIVITIES

JIM SLOAN

THE
MOUNTAINEERS

Published by
The Mountaineers
1001 SW Klickitat Way, Suite 201
Seattle, WA 98134

First edition, 1999

Published simultaneously in Great Britain by Cordee, 3a DeMontfort
Street, Leicester, England, LE1 7HD

Manufactured in Canada

Edited by Carol Anne Peschke
Cover and book design by Ani Rucki
Book layout by Alice C. Merrill

Cover photograph: © John Dick-TPI/Masterfile
Interior photopraphs: page 109 © digital STOCK; pages 9, 57, 93, 131,
157, 175, 201 © PhotoDisc™; pages 23, 145, 185 © Greg Mauer

Library of Congress Cataloging-in-Publication Data
Sloan, James, 1956–
    Staying fit over fifty / James Sloan. — 1st ed.
        p. cm.
    Includes bibliographical references and index.
    ISBN 0-89886-668-5 (pbk.)
    1. Physical fitness for the aged. 2. Physical fitness for middle aged
persons. 3. Exercise for the aged. 4. Exercise for middle aged persons. I. Trent, John. II. Title. III. Title: Staying fit over 50
    GV482.6 .s56 1999
    613.7'0446—dc21   99-6506
                                                         CIP

CONTENTS

PREFACE

Athletes talk of a moment in a race where the numbers don't match up with their sensations. They are going too fast to feel this good. The effort seems too easy, their movements unexpectedly graceful and light. They are like the triumphant runners of ancient Greece who became the "daimon," or spirit, and were allowed for a few moments to believe they shared in the gods' immortality. In that moment of easy speed and grace, you have manipulated time and space, found tight paths through physical laws and crumbling foundations.

But there is nothing mystical about it. You feel strong and graceful because in the weeks and months before this moment you have asked more of your body and it has responded. The body will always respond to physical stress by getting stronger. Your heart will get bigger and more powerful. Your blood will become richer, and it will push deeper into muscles that are working with calm precision, burning fat and sugar and clicking off contractions like well-oiled machines. It's not spiritual, it's science. It's engineering.

The purpose of this book is not to proselytize or preach the purity of purpose found in sport. You don't need to be told that again. Everybody from C. Everett Koop to Arnold Schwarzenegger has been hammering on that for some time now, and the studies showing the importance of exercise are being supplanted by studies showing that the real reason people don't exercise is because they don't like to be told what to do. So, for the record: I'm not telling you what to do. But I am telling you what happens when you do exercise and throwing in some suggestions on how to do it better as you get older.

My other goal is to reassure you. If you are at all like me—if you're in your forties, you've been active all your life, and you're wondering what kind of damage middle age will do to your fitness, speed, or flexibility— then I'm here to tell you that you have a lot to look forward to. Fitness is not a fountain of youth, but it certainly is a hedge against inflation. What I've learned researching and writing this book is that there is no reason for any of us to slow down or lower our expectations when it comes to fitness or general health; in fact, there are many reasons to look forward to aging and using exercise to conquer some of the many challenges we face in our lives—things like stress, doubt, and the muddled thinking that comes with working too hard and worrying that life is passing us by.

Who am I to talk? I'm nobody special. I am not Oprah's personal trainer or chef. I haven't invented any words like *aerobics* and I don't give lectures on fat and fitness for public television fundraisers. I'm not a scientist or a physiologist or a coach. I'm just someone like you, someone who was confused about conflicting reports on exercise and diet and set out to learn whether there were any simple truths left out there. I found that there are quite a few, and the simplest and truest thing I learned is this: The body will adapt. If you work it, it will find a way to work harder. If you rest it, it will repair itself and come back stronger than before.

If you are on the threshold of fifty, it's time to look at fitness in a new way. Understand it as a process, a thing that should be done with purpose, and let it work its magic for you. It is not an end in itself, but a means to an end, the end being the moments of clarity and self-assurance that follow a hard ski, a long run, or a challenging climb. There is no better time in life to accept another simple truth about exercise and fitness, and that is that the trick is not being the fastest or the strongest or having the most stamina. The trick is to make the most of what you've got. Most of us will never be champions; it's not that we don't work hard, it's just that we don't have the genetics. Once you've accepted that, the secret is to squeeze out as much horsepower as you can from that stock engine. Make it hum.

You can talk about the value of exercise in holding off disease and age, but there is more to it than that, more to it than I realized. Exercise makes you a more creative person, and more stable and independent and daring. These conclusions aren't drawn by New Age charlatans, but by scientists who have marveled at the capacity of older men and women who have stayed fit throughout their lives. Will you live longer if you exercise? Probably not. Will you live better? Will you sleep at night? Enjoy the flavor of your food? Yes, you will.

When we get busy, one of the first things we eliminate from our schedule is our workout. We'll skip it, trim it back, or scale it down to buy time. Sometimes that's to our advantage—some of us also forget that we need to take a day off from exercise once in a while—but most of the time it's a bankrupt way to act. We eliminate exercise to create time, but we are eliminating the one thing that can sharpen our senses and put things into the kind of perspective that can lead us to farsighted, intuitive solutions. If there is one thing I get preachy about, it's this: Respect your workout. Have faith that the time is well spent.

This book is based on the premise that if you understand why something works you are more likely to trust that it will work. There are still some secrets to be revealed about sport and fitness and how the human body responds to the physical demands we place on it, but we are talking about putting a gleam on the sharp edges. There aren't many big mysteries left. A personal trainer may help you get started or stay on an exercise program, but there isn't anything too complicated for you to figure out yourself, particularly if you use this book. As you'll learn reading it, the principles of training are fairly simple. And you can trust your body to let you know when you go astray. The secret, as with most things, is patience. As we approach our fiftieth birthdays, we come to believe we are on the precipice, that if we are to achieve our best it must be now or never. Don't make that mistake. Your best years are still in front of you.

For Karen,
Emma, and Lily

CHAPTER 1

UNDER-STANDING FITNESS

Rich Abrahams refuses to go gently into that good night. He's fifty-three years old, but he doesn't look it. And he certainly doesn't act it. He's just 6 feet tall, but he can jump from a stationary position and grab a basketball rim with both hands. He's a diligent weightlifter, and he's got the arms and shoulders to prove it. His voice has the timbre of that of a man twenty years younger.

But where Abrahams truly defies his age is in the swimming pool. He is the first person over age fifty to swim a 100-yard freestyle race in less than 50 seconds. If you don't know much about swimming, rest assured: That is fast—very fast. A lot of elite college swimmers would like to go that fast.

But what might be even more remarkable is that Rich Abrahams, at an age when most people are simply trying to hold onto what speed and strength they have, is getting faster. His time of 48.8 for the 100-yard freestyle is a full second faster than it was six years ago. His time for the 50-yard freestyle is actually faster than it was when he was in college thirty-five years ago.

"I don't really think about my age," he says. "I know I'm getting older and that eventually I'll slow down. But for now, I know there are a lot of things I can do to get faster. And that's what I intend to do—just keep getting faster."

In some ways, Rich Abrahams is typical of others in the vanguard of the Baby Boom generation; he refuses to accept long-held notions about the effects of aging. The population of Americans aged fifty and older will expand by nearly 50 million over the next twenty-five years, and many are entering middle age with dramatically different notions about aging than their parents and grandparents had. You might hear Abrahams moan a little bit as he hauls himself out of the pool at the end of a thunderous set of 100-yard repeats, and he'll say things like, "I'm getting too old for this stuff." But when you examine his expression you see the smirk, the irony. He's not getting too old for this. Not by a long shot.

And his attitude is shared by legions of older athletes around the world who are finding ways to stay fit and even get faster and stronger as they age. Some are exploiting new research that shows there are dozens of ways to offset the effects of age on our bodies, but even more are using their wisdom and experience to do things that only a generation ago scientists thought were impossible. Take John Hoffman as an example. He's one of the best rock climbers in the West, even though he's in his late fifties and has lost most of his climbing partners to more casual sports like golf and sailing. Twenty years ago a doctor might have told a guy John Hoffman's age to slow down, to conserve his energy because the heart has only so many beats and you don't want to waste them clinging to a granite overhang. But today, John Hoffman climbs with the kids, does laps on the tough indoor climbing wall he built in his house, and finds ways to work around the minor aches and pains that go with his passion. He leads tougher climbs today than he could twenty years ago, when he was supposed to be at the peak of physical prowess.

> AT AGE FIFTY-THREE, SWIMMER RICH ABRAHAMS IS GETTING *FASTER*.

And you're not going to hear him concede much to age.

"I know I'm not supposed to be as strong as I once was, but I'm climbing harder stuff," he says. "Maybe I'm just more savvy."

Call it what you will—strength, savvy, or just plain old staying power. Either way, Rich Abrahams, John Hoffman, and thousands of other athletes are putting some distance between themselves and Father Time. They've discovered something worth sharing.

A Booming Fitness Industry

The marketing experts tell us we Baby Boomers have built our identities on youth and vitality and that we're not about to let our fortieth or fiftieth birthdays change the way we think of ourselves. Maybe that's why fitness is a $3-billion industry in the United States. Membership in health clubs is soaring, attendance at community running races is up, and sales of in-home fitness equipment, from treadmills to cross-country ski simulators to stationary bikes, are increasing exponentially. In 1987, 4.4 million Americans exercised regularly on a treadmill. By 1997, 36 million did. Books such as Covert Bailey's *Fit or Fat* and *Smart Exercise*—folksy but at times highly technical looks at the physiological ramifications of diet and exercise—find a place on the best-seller lists. Dr. Kenneth Cooper, the man who coined the term *aerobics* and today is considered by many to be the father of the modern fitness boom, gives about fifteen speeches a month at $10,000–$15,000 a pop. Cooper has written fourteen books on fitness, and in 1997 he became a partner in a new $19-million fitness complex in Vero Beach, Florida, that will become the sister institute to his sprawling fitness research center in Dallas.

"We have developed a niche in medicine that, right now, is just exploding," Cooper says.

Never before, it seems, have Americans known so much about the benefits of exercise—how it can prolong life, stave off a wide variety

KEEPING YOUR MIND NIMBLE AND STRONG

While researchers are breaking new ground in studying physical aging, there is growing interest among scientists in changing long-held notions about how our minds age. According to one report, a revolution in attitude about aging is coming from an increasing number of scientists who want us to stop thinking age is an incurable disease that has to be treated with face-lifts and high-blood-pressure medicine. A team of European scientists is even attempting to define wisdom and characterize the patterns of insight and judgment that combine to create it.

Many of us come to believe that older people are frail, stubborn, and somewhat senile. We start developing these stereotypes at an early age and we grow old accepting them as the truth. And, accord-

ing to one theory, we live down to them. We see old age as a sexless, immobile, and decaying period of our lives.

But study after study has shown that if we respond creatively to change, look for ways to reduce anxiety, keep a positive outlook, and use our creative and inventive resources, we can keep our minds nimble and live longer. This is great news. Not only do we have new, solid evidence that we can maintain our physical prowess later in life, but we're also getting old at a time when society is increasingly aware of how wise we are. It's a great time to be getting older.

The men and women who are staying fit into their fifties are getting the most from their wisdom and physical strength. They have learned that fitness is not all about thundering heart rates

of deadly diseases, and keep your mental and physical faculties as sharp as a teenager's. Never before have people like Rich Abrahams had the knowledge and self-confidence it takes to swim 100 yards in less than 50 seconds. As recently as thirty years ago, physiologists believed you couldn't build muscle in an older person; now exercise experts are buying free weights for their grandmothers and ninety-year-olds are working out on weight machines in rest homes. Sixty-year-olds who are put on the same cardiovascular and strength-building programs as twenty-year-olds enjoy the same gains in muscle mass and endurance.

For generations we have believed that the body will slow down and dry up starting sometime after your thirty-fifth birthday. But now we know that isn't true. People who keep exercising won't see any

and buckets of lactic acid. It is about finesse, economy. It's about using your mind to squeeze a few extra horsepower from an engine that is already at maximum. You find that extra horsepower in technique and smart, analytical training. You find it in rest. You find it in diligence and method, but also in experimentation and spontaneity. You find it in the right application of your mental strength, concentration, and your sense of when to push it and when to back off.

The young ultramarathoners who go out on mountain runs with Joe Braninburg, a fifty-something contractor who has finished in the top ten at the 100-mile Western States Endurance Run, are often amazed at how quickly he moves across the rocky paths he trains on in the Sierra Nevada range outside his home in Reno. He doesn't look like he's running all that fast until you try to keep up with him. Then you realize how you are hopping over rocks and skidding down slopes while Braninburg is quietly moving over the terrain without any wasted effort. When you ask how he does it, he says, "Simply pick a line and follow it."

Easier said than done. But why should it be easy? Braninburg has been training for years. There has to be some advantage to his experience, and it is here, on these rocky traces at 9,000 feet, where it comes into play. Braninburg routinely beats guys twenty years younger, and it's not raw strength and VO_2 max that make the difference. It's his mental toughness, his experience, that makes the difference.

significant physical decline until they are sixty, and even then there is no reason to stop running or climbing mountains. Anything is possible. When you look at it this way, we are in a fitness renaissance, a turning point in history where science is flowing into mainstream attitudes to create a tide rich in health and promise.

The life expectancy of a typical American was forty-seven years in 1900; today it's around seventy-five and growing every year. In fifty years, the average life expectancy will be eighty-two years, and there will be more than 1 million people in the United States who are over one hundred years old. We are the beneficiaries of medical and social advancements that have nearly wiped out the threat of mass starvation, widespread homicide, unsanitary living conditions, and deadly epidemics. And we are growing old at a time when science has shown that the secret to living better and living longer is exercise. These are not charlatans telling us this. These are scientists.

It's Not All Downhill After Thirty-Five

Until recent years, most studies on aging were done on sedentary people. As people grew older you could document the decline in their strength and flexibility, the hardening of their arteries, the shortening of their breath and muscles. You could measure the thickening of their waists and hips, their increasing awkwardness, and the slow muddling of their minds. This was aging. People who exercised tended to skew the results, so they were left out.

That's changing. Scientists are showing more interest in studying how people like Rich Abrahams age, and what they are finding is quite amazing. In one study at the Center for Evaluation of Human Performance at Mount Sinai Medical Center in Milwaukee, a group of world-class athletes over age forty who continued to train and compete at high levels either maintained or improved their maximal oxygen consumption (VO_2 max) into their fifties. This flies in the face of previous findings that VO_2 max, the amount of oxygen a person can consume at the height of exercise, declines about 1 percent a year among sedentary people and 0.5 percent a year among fit people after their thirtieth birthday.

In fact, researchers found that those who continued to train hard didn't show much decline in general fitness until their late fifties and early sixties, and even then it was fairly minor. Elite athletes can't expect to continue to improve into their fifties because they trained at peak levels at a time early in life when their biological machinery was best suited to accommodate it. But for those of us who have stayed in shape but have been training inconsistently most of our lives, there is no reason why we can't use modern training theory and calculated approaches to get faster or stronger. Not only can we improve our fitness—our muscle strength and endurance, our aerobic capacity, our flexibility—but we can improve our times for a marathon or a 10-kilometer cross-country ski or a mile swim, at least until we're in our late fifties and sixties.

YOU CAN TEACH AN OLD DOG NEW TRICKS

Studies have shown that older people don't learn new sports as well as younger people do. There is often a physical reason for this: Sedentary people aren't as supple or strong as they once were and have lost reaction time as a result.

But even in forty- or fifty-year-olds who have stayed fit, the learning curve is a little steeper. A study in Sweden found that middle-aged golfers on a miniature golf course did worse than younger people when games were played with a soccer game broadcast in the background. Our ability to handle distractions like that declines with age.

Many older athletes may find the need or the desire to pick up a new sport later in life. This could happen if you get injured in your primary sport or just get the itch to try something new. If that's the case,

the secret will be to pick a sport similar to one you're already skilled at. You'll already have some neural grooves carved out. If you're a downhill skier, consider in-line skates, for instance.

Also, try visualization. Sit in a quiet spot and picture yourself doing the activity successfully. Picture a perfect conclusion. Researchers have found that blood rushes to the same areas of both the cortex (where conscious actions are regulated) and the cerebellum (where unconscious movements such as walking are stored), regardless of whether the athlete was performing or just thinking about their performance.

But above all else, practice. More and more, the movements of a new sport will be stored in the cerebellum. Practice makes perfect but it also makes it permanent.

A twenty-year study at the University of Southern California is finding that those who train and work hard can show impressive levels of fitness, even in advanced years. The study is tracking 150 competitive athletes who range in age from forty-something to ninety-one years old, with an average age of fifty-four. Every two years they come to a lab to run on a treadmill, get blood drawn, and get dunked in a body-fat–measuring water tank. It sounds pretty grueling, but most of the subjects in the study volunteered to be in it. Many of them run track and cross-country, but there are also cyclists, basketball players, and avid swing dancers in the group. One-fourth of the subjects are women—a group that has been neglected in other studies.

In addition to staying in great competitive shape—some of the athletes have lost only about 2 minutes a year in their marathon times—most of these people are also in excellent general health. Their levels of high-density lipoproteins (HDLs, the good cholesterol) are 40 to 60 percent higher than the average for people their age. Their pulse rates are much lower than average, and so is their blood pressure. They don't get sick as often. They want to live longer *and* healthier. Not all of them are elite athletes, but one thing they all share is that they have seen what is happening to other people their age and they don't want to have it happen to them.

Staying Motivated

Every day at around noon, Kim Layton, an estimator for an engineering firm who is in his late fifties, pulls away from his desk, drags out a small box filled with old running shoes, a wool hat, a paint-stained sweatshirt, and the rest of his workout clothes and heads out for a run along the river near his office. He runs 8 to 10 miles every day. When he returns, he quickly sponges off in the bathroom, puts his street clothes on, and gets back to work at his desk with a sandwich and a drink.

Layton has been an athlete for years. He was on the U.S. Olympic luge team in 1968. He's raced bicycles on a national level and he's pushed himself to the top ranks of cross-country skiers in his age group in recent years. He's an accomplished swimmer. And in 1998, his fifty-sixth year, he set a personal best in the marathon and achieved a goal he has sought for many years: He broke 3 hours for a 26.2-mile race. But there is nothing boastful or proud about this balding, white-haired man you see running through the railyards and past the factories near his office. There is a quiet, almost monastic devotion to his pursuits. And he doesn't think of age as an obstacle to his athletic pursuits.

"Age is only a number if you're willing to do something about it," he says.

You can talk at length about why some people (an estimated 22 percent of the country) stay with exercise programs and why most people who start exercising quickly drop out. They don't have time. They get injured. But the reason people like Kim Layton stay with exercise and continue to improve long after many have given up is more than plain determination. Kim Layton is an athlete. That is what he is. Being an athlete makes him happy. It makes him proud. He may not say that, but it does. The ancient Greeks, who asked the Persians to hold off their invasion until they were finished competing in their Olympic Games, called it their ethos—their guiding beliefs.

LEGIONS OF OLDER ATHLETES AROUND THE WORLD ARE FINDING WAYS TO STAY FIT AND EVEN GET FASTER AND STRONGER.

Patrick Fontane, a researcher from the St. Louis School of Pharmacology, has been studying older athletes for years. He's surveyed hundreds of older people who have not only stayed in shape but continued to compete in national events. Most of the people he talks to aren't champions—those seventy-year-old genetic aberrations who run a marathon a week—but regular folks who like to stay in shape and go to track-and-field or swim meets occasionally. The common thread he's found is that these people believe in and are motivated by what Fontane calls competitive health. When they go to the doctor, they want her to be shocked at how low their cholesterol levels are, how low their resting heart rate is, how voluminous their lungs are. About 55 percent of these people stay healthy because they want to compete; the rest compete because it helps them stay healthy.

And they want to prove something to themselves. This often

pushes them to remarkable achievements. The smart ones, according to Fontane, have "a sense of rhythm." They are more tuned into when it's time to push and when it's time to rest. And they find the time to work out.

"People come up with all sorts of excuses not to work out, but in the end it's about how you value your word to yourself," says Bari Beckett, a certified personal trainer, fitness video producer, and all-around high-powered fitness apostle. "It's about making a pact with yourself. You can't be committed to making a change with one foot out the door."

Writer John Jerome believes "staying with it," the title he chose for his book about returning to athletics in his late forties, requires "a leap of faith."

SUDDEN DEATH AND EXERCISE

Many people still hang onto the belief that vigorous exercise can kill you. Jim Fixx, the famous author and running advocate, died suddenly while jogging, and every few months, it seems, there are stories about supremely fit athletes dying unexpectedly. In one case, a fifty-seven-year-old American runner collapsed and died just a minute after setting a regional master's record for the 3,000 meters. Then there was the forty-two-year-old runner who had just missed breaking 3 hours in the marathon when he dropped dead. And Sergei Grinikov, a twenty-eight-year-old double Olympic gold medalist, died recently during a training run.

What the news stories about these tragedies don't explain is that most of these people would have died anyway, and that they probably would have died sooner if they hadn't been runners. A multitude of studies have shown that just about every athlete who dies suddenly during exercise has a serious disease, usually of the heart, and that none of their conditions is caused by exercise. In fact, the evidence is very clear that exercise hinders the development of many heart problems, particularly atherosclerosis.

But the sad truth is that you can be extremely fit and still have heart disease. Fixx, for instance, had severe coronary artery disease—one artery was completely plugged and another was 80 per-

"You have to believe in the training effect," he says. "The training effect is the astonishing physiological principle that says that the organism improves in response to stress. Every athlete has experienced its gentle galvanization. Athletes come to know that if they are only steadfast, the training effect will rescue them from torpor and temporary discomfort. Dropouts have to relearn this every time."

For most successful older athletes, there is a strong emotional component to their physical pursuits. A run, a climb, or a ski into the backcountry is a confluence of the body's work with the work of the mind. When we glance down at our watches and see that we have just run a mile faster than ever before and aren't even breathing hard yet, we have a sense that we have figured it out. The work is paying off. The heart is strong, the blood is rich, and the muscles are reliable and

cent blocked. Grinikov also had coronary artery disease. These runners, like many others, all had symptoms of heart disease—Fixx had very high blood cholesterol concentrations—but decided not to get them checked out.

Studies show that people who have advanced heart disease despite their training have an increased risk of dying during exercise. But if those people were to avoid exercise altogether, their overall risk of sudden death would increase, not decrease. Some studies have found that moderate exercise does not increase the risk of sudden death in those with advanced heart disease and other studies have shown that more vigorous exercise—such as running and cross-country skiing—is associated with a 5 to 7 times greater risk of sudden death.

If you're fit but still have symptoms of a heart problem or a family history of heart problems, you need to consult a doctor before continuing any hard training. In fact, anyone over fifty who wants to start exercising should get a cardiovascular screening first. Medical researchers say many people with heart disease can exercise without risking sudden death. If you're already exercising and start to feel chest pains or other symptoms, back off and see a doctor immediately. Although the incidence of heart disease in athletes is rare—anywhere from 1 in 10,000 to 1 in 200,000—it's a mistake to think you're safe just because you're fit.

willing to do the work. Psychologists say that most people are unhappy because they rush about too much. They worry about what happened this morning while they anticipate what will happen this afternoon. They overlook the here and now, the moment, the liberating pleasure of a bite of food or a sip of cold water on a hot day. This is what sport—exercise—gives back to older athletes. It brings us back to the moment in which we are living and it sharpens its joys and sorrows—just as light rays are gathered in a lens and focused into heat and flame.

Sport forces you to reclaim your body, to reoccupy its outer reaches. Gerontologists tell us that people who are sedentary lose touch with their bodies—they feel broader and heavier than they really are, and activities feel harder than they should be. They aren't sure where their

WHY ARE WE SO FAT?

Dozens of surveys have been conducted in recent years in an effort to gauge just how fit the United States is, and none has been very promising. The *Journal of the American Medical Association (JAMA)* estimates that 33 percent of American adults are overweight, and the Institute of Medicine reported in 1995 that 59 percent of the American population is too heavy. There have been other estimates, but most experts agree that at least half the nation is over-weight and that one in four meets the definition for clinical obesity, defined as 20 percent above ideal body weight.

And people aren't kidding themselves; a survey by the Calorie Control Council, a nonprofit association of companies that manufacture low-calorie foods, revealed that 60 percent of Americans feel they need to lose weight. And by almost any measure, the number of fat folk in our land is increasing—the *JAMA* study estimates that obesity has increased 25 percent since the 1960s.

When you look at all the studies done on exercise, you can see why. One study found that only 22 percent of Americans are doing any kind of meaningful exercise. When the Centers for Disease Control surveyed 106,000 adults in all fifty states in 1994, it found that 30 percent of the country does nothing—no walking, no golf, not even any gardening. *Prevention* magazine does an annual index of America's health habits, and each year it gets about the same result: Only 37 percent of American adults are doing enough work to gain aerobic benefits. The numbers decline as people age; less

bodies end, and it makes them tentative, clumsy. But humans, psychologist Dan Dervin says, have a need to "stimulate the sense of inner aliveness." We're the only species that's like that. Those who train talk of feeling their bodies stretching out, of feeling their senses of smell and taste sharpen. "One of the most immediate benefits of training was the fine, loose feeling of inhabiting my whole body again," says Jerome of the time he spent training for an attempt to set an age-group record for the 1,650-yard freestyle swim. That's a great feeling.

"Sports' true and lasting victory is over the numbness that comes from fear or boredom or over the deadness that comes from being helpless or inert," Dervin says. "Perhaps we have after all now struck the nerve of motive."

---

than 10 percent of those over sixty-five engage in any strenuous exercise.

These distressing numbers come despite an all-out effort by several health organizations to get Americans exercising. Scientists have published study after study showing that inactivity leads to heart disease, diabetes, colon cancer, high blood pressure, obesity, osteoporosis, joint problems, and general malaise. Exercise is the only way to counter all these problems. Consequently, everybody from the Public Health Service, which wants to reduce America's sedentary ranks to 15 percent, to the American College of Sports Medicine, which has devised a user-friendly exercise pyramid to help people understand how much they should exercise, is trying to get the word out. But it's not working.

The problem, the experts agree, is that messages are mixed. When scientists recommended that people accumulate their exercise over the course of the day in short bursts—a strategy devised to get people doing something—many misinterpreted the advice and thought walking to the coffee pot ten times a day was as good as a 30-minute jog. Another problem is the public's unrealistic expectations about exercise. The image of fitness created by the exercise industry emphasizes lean, sculpted bodies, and when people start an exercise program and don't get bulging muscles, they figure they are wasting their time and quit.

The cost? As many as a quarter of a million Americans are dying every year

(Continued on next page)

because they consume far more calories than they burn up in exercise. Epidemiologists at Harvard University estimate that treating obesity and the diabetes, heart disease, high blood pressure, and gallstones caused by it accounted for $45.8 billion in health care costs in 1990, the latest year studied. Indirect costs because of missed work contributed another $23 billion. All of these costs have a direct bearing on your insurance premiums and your income.

America's inertia has experts scratching their heads. Here you have millions of people faced with the prospect of living longer than many ever dreamed possible.

And they know that the one thing that they can do to forestall every effect of aging is to exercise. But hardly any of them are doing it.

It seems Americans will do anything to fight fat except exercise. According to a 1994 congressional study, Americans spent about $33 billion that year on weight-loss products and services, many of which have only short-term benefits if they help at all. Many of these programs boast that you can drop weight without doing any exercise, ignoring careful scientific research that shows the only way to take weight off and keep it off is through a combination of diet and exercise.

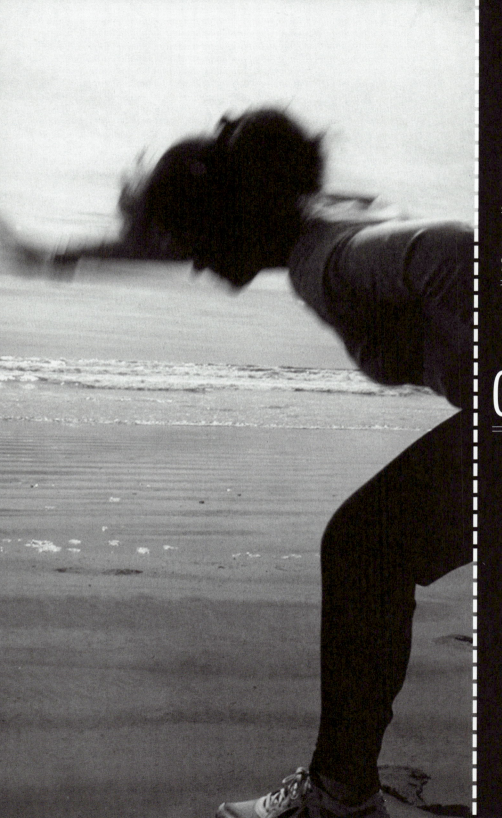

CHAPTER 2

EXERCISE AND THE EFFECTS OF AGING

Nikki Rippee, an expert on aging who teaches at the University of Nevada, Reno, keeps a series of photographs in her office to show her students what they've got to look forward to as they get older.

The photographs show a man—a weightlifter—at the end of each decade of his life. There's a photo of him at thirty, one at forty, and so on into his sixties. It's a sobering picture. It's humbling. But not for the reason you might think.

YOU CAN SLOW THE EFFECTS OF AGE, BUT IT TAKES SOME WORK.

From decade to decade, you can barely see any change in the man. You can see he's getting older—his hair is thinning and those wisdom lines around his eyes become more etched as time goes on—but his body hardly changes at all. "Maybe you see a little decline in muscle mass after his sixtieth birthday, but you have to look hard," Rippee says. "People don't realize that our idea of aging is changing. You don't have to grow old like you used to. But it takes some work."

That's the humbling part. The man in the poster didn't put the brakes on time just by having good genes. He worked at it.

Even in this day of antiaging creams, face-lifts, and liposuction, aging usually isn't a pretty sight. We're used to seeing people slide into a steady rate of decline as they get older. Their muscles shrink, their shoulders and back stoop, and their bones get thin and weak. They lose their balance and flexibility. Their blood pressure goes up as their arteries harden. Their skin gets loose and their minds start to go. Scientists call this homeostenosis, the declining ability of the aging body to adapt to physical stresses and demands. Left untouched—just fed and watered and used for routine tasks—the human body very steadily shrinks, curls up, gets brittle, and wheezes along with an increasingly perceptible limp.

Unless, of course, you stay in shape.

"The rate of decline for an active person is really much more stately than we ever thought before," says Walter Bortz, a gerontologist with the Palo Alto Medical Foundation.

Bortz should know. Although he's in his late sixties, he can run a marathon in just over 4 hours. His wife ran the 100-mile Western States

Endurance Run at age sixty in just over 24 hours—a time a lot of young guys never achieve.

Stave Off the Effects of Age

Scientists estimate that a sedentary man—because of muscle loss, a decreasing maximum heart rate (MHR), and stiffening lungs and arteries—loses about 10 percent of his ability to do work every decade after age thirty-five. What does that mean, exactly? Well, if your best time for an all-out mile run at age thirty-five is 6 minutes, your best time for an all-out run thirty years later will be almost 8 minutes. What was once an easy jog will become a lung-searing effort.

But with exercise and smart training, you can cut your losses dramatically. Take a look at a measurement known as VO_2 max, which is the maximum amount of oxygen you use while exercising at your limit for 1 minute. Physiologists determine your VO_2 max by putting you on a treadmill and measuring how much oxygen you are using as you exercise. If you are well trained, your muscles will use a lot of oxygen for energy and your heart will be big and strong and capable of pushing a lot of oxygen-rich blood deep into those working muscles. You'll have a high VO_2 max reading. If you're unfit, your muscles won't have many oxygen-burning enzymes and will tire before much oxygen is put to work.

Sedentary people lose what VO_2 max they have at a rate of about 10 percent per decade. That's because your MHR decreases, the amount of blood your heart pulls in and pushes out decreases, and your arteries become less elastic, increasing your blood pressure as your body struggles to force blood through the body.

But most fit people don't have these problems. Recent studies show they lose VO_2 max at a rate of only 0.5 percent a year—sometimes even less. In one study, a group of fifty-six-year-old runners with similar training habits and race times were compared with a carefully matched group of twenty-five-year-old runners, and the difference in VO_2 max was only 9 percent, or 0.3 percent per year. In yet another study, older runners between the ages of fifty and eighty-two who had maintained training volumes and intensities over a ten-year period showed no decrease in VO_2 max. The only reason some athletes lose VO_2 max is because their MHRs decrease with age, something no amount of training can change.

EXERCISE AND HEART ATTACKS

Although extremely fit people sometimes have heart attacks and die, the truth is that vigorous exercise does much more to prevent heart attacks than to cause them. Exercise lowers your blood pressure and resting heart rate, thus reducing your risk of a heart attack.

Although the research is not conclusive at this point, it seems that exercise encourages the metabolism of cholesterol so that less is floating around in the blood looking for something to attach itself to. Exercise also seems to increase the percentage of high-density lipoproteins (HDLs) found in your blood. HDLs, unlike low-density lipoproteins (LDLs), keep cholesterol moving through the blood without grabbing hold of the inner walls of the arteries and damming things up. That blockage is known as atherosclerosis, and accounts for 30 percent of all deaths each year. A 1996 study in the *New England Journal of Medicine* found that HDL levels increased in women as they increased the amount they were running each week. Women who ran more than 64 kilometers a week (36 miles) had significantly higher concentrations of HDL than women who ran less than 48 kilometers.

Of course, a lack of exercise is just one of the factors that leads to thrombosis (the complete blockage of an artery) and angina (the shortness of breath and chest pain that precede a heart attack). The other factors include smoking, excessive weight gain, a high-fat diet, and stress. It's no coincidence that people who exercise usually don't have any of these other problems either.

What do you have to do to achieve higher HDL levels and decrease your cholesterol? According to fitness expert and scientist Covert Bailey, you have to exercise at 65 to 80 percent of your MHR for 30 or 40 minutes, 3 to 4 days a week. That's a pretty tough workout schedule, but the payoff is high.

Recent research indicates there may be other ways that exercise protects the heart. According to a study at the University of South Carolina, exercise increases the level of a heart-protecting enzyme called tissue plasminogen activator (TPA). TPA is produced by the inner lining of the blood vessels for the purpose of breaking up clots in the bloodstream. In fact, a genetically engineered version of TPA is

And here's another thing to keep in mind: No matter how old you are, you can always improve your aerobic capacity. Elderly people put on an exercise program show the same increases in VO₂ max as young

used as medicine for heart attack victims, 90 percent of whom suffered their attacks because of clots. The study also found that exercise dramatically decreased levels of a plasminogen activator inhibitor (PAI-1), which binds to TPA and renders it useless.

The study examined three groups of fifteen men. One group did no exercise, the second group ran about 30 minutes a day 3–5 days a week, and the third group was composed of competitive runners who worked out an hour a day five or more times a week. They were all between age twenty-six and forty-three.

Although they all had similar levels of TPA at rest, all three groups showed increases in TPA after doing a treadmill test of 11–15 minutes that took them to exhaustion. The sedentary men doubled their levels of TPA but the exercising group had sharply higher increases. What's more, PAI-1 levels at rest—which were highest for nonexercisers—dropped even further after the workout: 19 percent for the sedentary group and 51 percent for the elite athlete group.

What does it all mean? For starters it explains why fit people are less likely to have heart attacks than sedentary people. Not only do they have stronger hearts, lower body fat, and better circulation, but their blood chemistry is also working to keep the system flowing smoothly. The study also suggests that exercise trains blood vessels to respond to stress just as it trains muscles to respond. However, researchers were quick to point out that the tests were limited and needed to be expanded. How much do increases in TPA help the blood and the heart? Is the effect the same in men older than fifty-five, whose heart attack risks are higher? And what about women? No doubt we'll be hearing more about TPA in the future.

These and other findings underscore the value of exercise for anyone. The cardiopulmonary system responds to training no matter how little exercise you've done in your life. Some folks who have stayed fit can use exercise to dramatically improve their heart and lung functions, and some people taking on a fitness program for the first time will see a quick and substantial improvement in the health of their hearts. That's a fountain of youth.

unfit people put on the same program. There is even evidence to discredit the long-held notion that older people need more time to progress and adapt to endurance training.

Women don't lose VO$_2$ max at the same rate men do. Women typically have lower VO$_2$ maxes to begin with, but the difference between the two sexes decreases as time marches on, some researchers say. This could be one reason why so many older women seem more vital than their husbands later in life.

In a 1993 study, researchers put a group of sedentary men and women between the ages of sixty and sixty-five years on a nine-month training program. Both groups increased their aerobic capacity by 20 percent, but they went about it in different ways. The men developed bigger hearts that pumped more blood. But the women, with their smaller, less adaptive hearts, got their fitness gains by developing more capillaries (the twigs of the blood-delivery branches) and more mitochondria in their muscles.

Walter Bortz looked at the effects of aging from another angle. He analyzed performance data for running, rowing, and swimming events from national organizations, plotted winning times according to age

HOW MUCH WILL I SLOW DOWN?

Many older athletes find that even while they are maintaining endurance, they still lose some speed and don't recover from hard workouts as fast as they once did.

The American Running and Fitness Association suggests older runners do long runs only every two or three weeks, for instance, and reduce their hard speed work to just once a week or every other week. Famous running author George Sheehan ran only three times a week—

two 10-milers and a weekend race—when he was at top form and winning his age group in local races.

Aging has widely varied effects on people. Most runners who could finish a marathon in 3 hours when they were younger find their times increasing to 3:30 as they enter their sixties. Others lose only a couple of minutes a year. Then there are guys like New Zealander Derek Turnbull, who cranked out a phenomenal 2:38 in his sixties. Some ex-

groups after age thirty-five, and found that curves for all three sports followed the same slope. After comparing these results with other physiological markers, such as VO$_2$ max, he concluded that the rate of decline for extremely physically fit people is just 5 percent per decade. "Anything more than that," Bortz said, "must be due to inactivity."

Another researcher, Stephen Seiler in Norway, suggests that the decline in VO$_2$ max in hard-charging master athletes who aren't yet fifty might be even less: on the order of 1 to 2 percent per decade after age twenty-five.

So if you can run a 6-minute mile in your thirties and you keep training hard into your sixties, what will your mile time be when you're sixty-five? Well, if it's true that you don't lose much of anything until you're fifty and that after that the decrease is 0.5 percent annually, you should be able to run that mile in 6:27.

Not bad for a senior citizen.

What Is It About Exercise That Helps?

If your VO$_2$ max is high, it means your heart is strong, your lungs and arteries are accommodating and elastic, and your muscles are lean,

perts theorize that athletes who are also very physically active in their everyday lives—such as the Tamahumara Indians of Mexico—don't slow down as much as recreational athletes from industrialized societies. Turnbull, it should be noted, is a farmer who works hard all day in his fields.

Runners may find that their performance declines faster in marathon distances than it does in 10-kilometer or half-marathon distances. Anecdotal evidence indicates that some older runners' marathon times balloon by 25 percent in their sixties while their shorter-distance times increase by only 10 or 15 percent. But these are athletes who have trained at a high level all their lives. If you've always been a runner but have never seriously done interval training, you may find your times dropping in your fifties and sixties if you add some purposeful speed work to your weekly training schedule.

hungry, and ready to burn oxygen to create energy and power for contractions. Some of that is hereditary, but exercise helps. An average sedentary man in his mid-thirties will have a VO_2 max of 40–45 milliliters of oxygen per minute per kilogram of body weight. That same man can increase his VO_2 max to 50–55 milliliters per minute per kilogram with an endurance training program. The exercise trains all the elements of the fitness equation, right down to the body's cellular and chemical functions. To give you a better idea of how all this works, let's look at how training benefits your heart, lungs, muscles, bones, and nervous system—all the elements that contribute to how fast you'll run that mile.

How the Heart Adapts to Training

The heart is a muscle and it responds to the stresses of training as any other muscle does: It gets stronger. The heart is a muscular balloon, and when you exercise, the balloon is filled by the extra blood being squeezed back into it by exercising muscles. The heart has to work harder to push the extra blood back out to the body, and in that process it gets stronger. When the pressure is off, your heart beats slower and stronger, fueling the body with fewer beats than before it became trained. At rest, a typical sedentary person's heart beats 70 times a minute, pushing out about 70 milliliters per beat. But after three months of endurance training, an average person's resting heart rate may decrease to 55 beats per minute. At the same time, his or her stroke volume might increase to 90 milliliters.

Although your MHR will decline, your advancing age should not diminish your hard-won stroke volume if you continue to work out. Your heart will be as big as a younger opponent's, and much larger than that of another person the same age who doesn't work out. Keep in mind that stroke volume is hard to measure and not all researchers agree that you can maintain the same volume as you age. But one thing is clear: If your volume is maintained, it's probably because all that exercise you are doing is helping keep your arteries supple so the blood can move more easily through the body. Exercise also increases your number of capillaries, which take the blood from vessels and distribute it to the muscles.

Strengthening Muscles and Bones

We've all had sore muscles before. You wake up after your first good cross-country ski workout and your back and shoulders feel like gremlins have been pounding them with little hammers all night. How does the muscle respond to the abuse you heaped on it? By getting stronger. Although researchers aren't sure what causes muscle soreness—whether it is caused by small tears or free radicals or something else—they do know that the muscle, after it's repaired, becomes more resistant to injury and learns to repair itself faster from future gremlin attacks. And that does not change as you age. Studies have shown that even sedentary people in their eighties and nineties can vastly improve their muscular strength with resistance training.

Men start losing muscle after age twenty-five, and the rate of decline is about 7 pounds a decade if they don't do anything to halt this withering process. Both the size and number of muscle fibers decrease after age thirty, and the fast-twitch group is especially hard hit. You may not notice a loss of strength until after age forty, but you'll lose 5 percent of your strength every decade after that. Unless you recruit your fast-twitch fibers (that is, do sprints), there is evidence that you'll start losing those motor units at the rate of 10 percent a decade after age fifty. This means that a twenty-five-year-old man who weighs about 170 pounds and has about 89 pounds of muscle will lose 14 pounds of lean body mass—mostly muscle—by the time he's forty-five. His metabolic rate will decline accordingly, and if his caloric intake is not reduced at the same rate, his body fat will increase dramatically. He might weigh the same twenty years later, but he won't look the same.

According to one study in 1981, most people gain 0.2–0.8 kilograms of fat a year after ages twenty to thirty, which means there are a lot of people tripling their body fat by the time they reach age sixty. Women who don't exercise and do strength work lose about 5 pounds of muscle a decade after age thirty-five, and after menopause the losses accelerate to about a pound a year.

You can head off most of these changes—and even get stronger—with regular upper- and lower-body strength training. After age sixty, however, both testosterone and growth hormone seem to drop more dramatically, and muscle fibers begin to atrophy. But your losses in strength won't be as great if you continue to lift weights into your sixties.

Working a muscle encourages the body to push more capillaries into the fibers of that muscle. This increases the flow of blood, oxygen, and fuel into the working muscle. You don't lose this ability as you age; in fact, one study showed that fit older runners had the same number of capillaries in their running muscles as much younger runners. An ex-

LIVING A LONG LIFE

Barring unforeseen circumstances—like pneumonia or a heart attack—the reasons we die can be traced to three processes within the body. The first is genetic and the second two are chemical.

All cells, whether in turtles or humans, reproduce only a certain number of times. After that, their metabolism fades and their skin collapses and they die. We don't know why and we don't know how to stop it. And until we do it's likely that everyone—even a hundred-year-old marathoner who always practiced safe sex—will die by age one hundred twenty years.

But what takes most of us well before then are two chemical reactions in our body. One involves free radicals, the detritus left over from energy production. This gunk of oxygen molecules binds to anything it can find, weakening internal tissues and organs and sometimes leading to cancer. The body can fight off the ravages of free radical oxidation only so long before it caves in.

The other reaction is called glycosyl-ation. That's where sugar bonds with protein and causes things to plug up: joints, arteries, the lenses of the eye. The process is very similar to the browning that occurs in cooking, and there isn't much you can do to prevent it.

Although scientists haven't perfected free radical therapies and drugs to counter the effect of glycosylation, there is still hope for those who want to live a very, very long life. All they have to do is cut their calorie intake to near-starvation levels.

Clive McCay, a scientist at Cornell in the 1930s, found that he could extend the life of mice by 50 percent by cutting their diets way, way back, so that they barely had enough to live. Later researchers learned that putting other animals on scant but nutritious diets not only prolonged their lives but kept them youthful into a very old age.

Roy L. Walford, a professor of pathology at the University of California, Los Angeles, took up where McCay left off and

ercised muscle will also increase its number of mitochondria, the little energy factories the muscle needs to produce fuel for contractions. Mitochondria increase your aerobic capacity and reduce your rate of lactic acid production. But if the training stops, the mitochondria slowly disappear; in sedentary people, activity in the muscles' mitochondria—as measured by the enzymes that do the work—declines 25 to 40 percent as they get older.

has found that these spare diets improve an animal's immune system, lower blood pressure and cholesterol, and reverse arteriosclerosis. Cancer in these animals is rare. Walford, age seventy-one, got such good results from so many different animals that he put himself on the diet and now plans to live another half-century. His book, *The Anti-Aging Plan,* includes more than 100 recipes that are primarily vegetarian.

Walford was one of eight researchers who followed the diet while living in Biosphere 2. The men lost 33 pounds on average and the women who followed the diet lost 17 pounds. Their cholesterol and blood pressure readings all went down, too. The only drawback to the diet, it seems, was that the dieters had recurring and elaborate fantasies about the food they were being denied.

Why does near starvation help? It probably decreases the production of free radicals by decreasing the amount of food being burned up by your cells and lowering your body temperature by a degree or two.

If you can't picture yourself reducing your caloric intake 30 percent, here's hope: Gerontologists with the National Institute on Aging's Gerontology Research Center in Baltimore say a drug may be developed to allow you to eat but still gain the benefits of starvation. But that drug is still twenty years away.

If you're impatient for a sip from the fountain of youth, you might try hormone replacement therapy. This therapy counters the effects of menopause—and estrogen losses that accompany it—and has been shown to increase life expectancy by eight years, particularly among women who have one or more risk factors for heart disease. The hormone therapy can also prevent colon cancer, reduce wrinkling, and keep your teeth strong. The therapy apparently can help men, but most don't want to put up with the side effects, such as increased breast size.

And there's no reason why you can't keep those muscles as limber as they were when you were younger. Although time tends to tighten us up—our muscles shorten as the elastin and collagen in our connective tissues become frayed and more dense—there is reason to believe that this effect can be delayed. When researchers put a group of teenagers in a stretching program with a group of seniors between the ages of sixty-three and eighty-eight, both groups saw the same improvement in flexibility after six weeks. The price you pay for not stretching becomes more severe with age; your flexibility can decline as much as 30 percent, shortening your stride and forcing you to work harder to maintain the same speed you once took for granted.

Bones respond to stress the same way muscles do: by getting stronger. Although lifting weights and exercising can't make bones any denser than they naturally are, they can offset the slow decline that starts to affect women after age thirty-five and men after age fifty.

Osteoporosis is a chronic and often crippling condition caused by thin, brittle bones. It affects an estimated 25 million Americans, mostly white women over age sixty, and is the twelfth leading cause of death in the United States. More than 700,000 fractures a year among women are linked to osteoporosis.

Our bones are metabolically active, building and rebuilding themselves with the nutrients we give them. Collagen fibers form a web throughout the bone and such minerals as calcium, phosphorus, sodium, magnesium, copper, chloride, potassium, zinc, iron, and manganese attach to that mesh. Bones need constant nourishment to carry out this work.

A woman's bone mass peaks in her late twenties or early thirties and starts to wane by age forty. The rate of bone loss, left unchecked, increases when women reach age fifty and their estrogen levels decrease during menopause. At this point, the mineral content of the bones declines and bones become thinner and weaker. It usually reaches a critical stage for sedentary women at age sixty. Some women's upper spines bend and bulge into a "dowager's hump" just below the neck.

A July 1998 study published in the *Annals of Internal Medicine* found that the more active a woman is, the less likely she is to break a hip.

Those who benefit the most are the women doing more vigorous stuff like aerobic dance, tennis, and weightlifting. Even fit women who run or walk benefit from adding upper-body resistance training to their workouts.

The Nervous System

Your ability to send and receive neural messages diminishes as you age and results in slower reaction time—probably by about 10 percent slower after the age of fifty. That's why major league baseball players usually don't stay in the game longer. We also experience a decline in sensory perception, such as hearing and vision, because the brain doesn't use glucose as well as we age. This all adds up to losses in agility, balance, and coordination.

INDIVIDUALS WHO TRAIN BECOME MORE SELF-CONFIDENT, PRECISE, AND PERSISTENT.

But the exercise you're doing can keep all these changes at bay. Studies have shown that training increases the blood flow to the cerebral region, and that alone helps improve coordination, balance, and overall readiness. Studies in the late 1980s confirmed that aerobic exercise could also improve an aging person's visual organization, memory, and mental flexibility. That's because exercise postpones structural changes in the nerve cell and the loss of dendrites in the aging brain.

How Fitness Can Redefine Aging

In many ways, those of us who exercise are helping change the way the world looks at aging. For years researchers have had a hard time determining what changes to the body are caused by aging and which ones are caused by inactivity. The decreases in physical ability that we've always associated with aging also show up in healthy astronauts sent into space for an extended period of time. It also happens to athletes who get injured and are forced to rest in bed. They lose strength, flexibility, and stamina. Their blood pressure goes up and so does their resting heart rate. Their muscles shorten and their bones weaken.

The constrictions of age—the decreased range of motion in the joints, the shortening of muscles and breath, the increased pressure within as blood pushes against stiffening passageways—are in many ways a metaphor for what happens to the mind and personality of an unfit person as he or she ages. Studies that go back more than twenty years have found that middle-aged men who never exercise lose some of their physical courage. They fear more for their health and safety, and there is more tension in their lives. They tend to become introverted. Increasingly, it seems, they fall into the role society has carved out for them and they become tentative, cautious, maybe even a little suspicious.

Those who train, on the other hand, become more self-confident, precise, and persistent. They take on big projects and they aren't crippled by the prospect of failure. They are better at relaxing, possibly because of the "natural opiates" of enkephalin and beta-endorphin released by hard exercise, but more likely because their fitness gives them a sense of accomplishment. That's no small thing in a world like ours where the results of our professional work are often fleeting and evanescent. There has been a debate going on for more than two decades over whether running improves someone's mental health. Some say there is a direct link; others argue there is just the appearance of one because runners are taking a break from the day's stress and gaining mastery over time and their body. If the result is the same, who cares?

According to a Harvard University study, women who run produce a less potent form of estrogen than sedentary women, which cuts their risk of breast or uterine cancer in half. Other studies show that exercise does not reduce the risk of breast cancer in younger women but may play a role in protecting postmenopausal women from the disease.

Will exercise help us live longer? It's hard to say. There are a lot of factors that affect our lifespans: Medical advances will help keep us alive, as will our own native curiosity about life and our keen interest in continuing our enjoyment of it. A Harvard alumni study published in *JAMA* in April 1995 concluded that vigorous exercise, like running, "helps to prolong the lives of middle-aged men," but easy stuff like gardening won't keep you around longer. Perhaps the only thing you can say with certainty is that the quality of your life will improve if you stay fit: You will stay strong and active later in life, you won't get sick as often, and you're less likely to wind up in a hospital in your later years. You will sleep better. Your food will taste better.

Ironically, studies show that people who live a long time tend to be people who don't give much thought to living a long time. Unlike the Struldbruggs—the people in *Gulliver's Travels* who obsessed about their immortality and went slowly insane because of it—modern-day nonagenarians think less about the length of life than they do about the content of life. They read and take classes. They exercise because they want to continue to enjoy the things they love: hikes into the mountains, swims in cold alpine lakes. They keep their minds nimble and engaged.

They stay alive.

MENOPAUSE

The first of 38 million female Baby Boomers has just turned fifty-two, one year after the average age of menopause, and doctors' offices are filling up with women in their forties complaining of hot flashes, insomnia, unpredictable bleeding, and mood swings. These women are experiencing perimenopause, the period of declining estrogen levels that leads up to the time when they stop menstruating altogether. An increasing number are turning to their doctors for hormone treatments and other drugs to alleviate their symptoms.

Although doctors rarely used to prescribe estrogen before menopause, many are handing out pills and patches for women in their thirties and forties, despite studies showing that long-term use raises the risk of breast and uterine cancer. There is also growing concern in the medical world that doctors are wrongly medicalizing what for centuries has been a natural transition that causes most women little or temporary discomfort. Doctors argue that if it makes people feel better, why not use it? However, most doctors are quick to tell their patients that proper diet and exercise are a good treatment for many of the symptoms of perimenopause, including hot flashes and insomnia.

Women who are approaching menopause, even those who increase their exercise and improve their eating habits, find that they get thicker and heavier. It starts in your mid-thirties and keeps going until your mid-forties. It's a time in which metabolism slows down and muscle slowly converts to fat. What's happening is that as you approach age forty, you start producing less estrogen. And because estrogen is produced in the fat cells, the fat cells get bigger in an effort to maintain production. And these larger fat cells, which congregate around your waist because those are the cells that are best equipped to produce estrogen, are more resistant to dieting.

Ironically, these fat cells help you out once you reach menopause. According to Debra Waterhouse, the author of *Outsmarting the Midlife Fat Cell,* these fat cells help control hot flashes, mood swings, and PMS. They also help you sleep better during menopause and reduce the risk of osteoporosis.

Does that mean you should leave the weight on? No. Waterhouse says you can lose some of the weight while still holding off the effects of menopause. She suggests doing aerobic exercise and strength-building workouts and eating a wide variety of foods, including fruits, vegetables, and foods high in protein and calcium.

Waterhouse has studied menopausal women for nearly twenty years and has found that those who survive menopause with the least amount of discomfort have these seven habits:

- They don't worry about weight loss, but about body composition (percentage of body fat). Forget weight-loss clinics and throw out your scale. Pinch your skin to see whether you are losing fat.
- They have accepted their bodies. If they are pear-shaped and stocky, they don't expect to be tall and lanky.
- They exercise for at least an hour at least 4 days a week at mode rate levels. And they do a variety of activities, from jogging and swimming to in-line skating and aerobic dance.
- They drink water throughout the day.
- They eat every few hours to keep blood sugar stable and moods tempered.
- They eat their big meal at lunch and lightest meal in the evening, when caloric needs of a menopausal woman drop off dramatically.
- They still enjoy their favorite foods.

Many experts agree that the top priority for postmenopausal women is exercise. Doctors often prescribe estrogen supplements as well, and many women are exploring unproven nutritional supplements such as soy powder, wild yam, red clover, black cohosh, chasteberry, don quai, licorice root, yarrow, motherwort, and milk thistle. Studies of women in Asia indicate that soy products may help relieve menopausal symptoms, although most doctors will tell you more study is needed.

CHAPTER 3

THE TRAINING EFFECT

When doctors wanted to find out how people adapt to exercise, they put some untrained guys on a treadmill, set the speed at 7 miles an hour, and watched as they gasped and sweated through a timed workout. Then they pulled them into a lab, drew some blood, and tested how much lactic acid was swirling around in there.

There was quite a bit.

PUSHING YOURSELF, EVEN A LITTLE, YIELDS BIG GAINS ON THE FITNESS FRONT.

It's no secret that lactic acid stalks the blood of the unfit like Dracula prowls around looking for rosy virgins. Lactic acid forms in the muscle and seeps into the bloodstream during exercise when our muscles demand more energy than our bodies can produce by burning fat with oxygen. We switch over to burning sugar exclusively and that's when the trouble starts. Before long, our muscles start to feel heavy, then start to sting, and then our body, without much debate at all, simply slows down all by itself. We start to feel clumsy and then we have to stop altogether.

And that was the case for these poor guys in this study.

But what's interesting is that over the next 10 days, while they exercised at the same pace as that first day, their lactic acid concentration slowly declined until it finally leveled off. It stayed at the same concentration for the next ten daily workouts, at a level that was about half what it started out as. What was happening was that the test subjects were getting in shape by learning how to burn fat better. So the researchers did what any self-respecting physiologists would do: They cranked up the speed to 8.5 miles an hour.

The result? Lactic acid levels soared again then dropped steadily over the next several days before leveling off again. The runners' reliance on sugar declined as their affection for aerobic energy—energy created by burning fat—increased. After nearly two months, the blood lactate levels were about one-fifth what they had been when the test started and the subjects were running 7-minute miles with greater ease than they'd run 8.5-minute miles at the start of the test.

The body is a resilient organism. It adapts. If we overwork a muscle and make it sore and damaged, it will repair itself and come back stronger and more likely to withstand future stress. The essence of exercise and fitness programs is to create a need for more aerobic energy by working longer and harder than your body is used to. Then you give it the nutrients it needs to repair itself and give it time to do the repairs. And then you start all over again. Only this time your muscles are just a little stronger, so you have to work out a little harder. And then a little harder.

Coaches call it the principles of overload and progression, and it's how people steadily get stronger and faster and gain endurance. In theory, it is the process of slowly and methodically stressing your body beyond its ability to comfortably provide energy for the work you're doing. In practice, it's the process of diligently bringing down your times for those mile repeats you do on the track every Wednesday morning. You are asking more of your body: your muscles, heart, lungs, and circulatory system. And they all adapt. It's called the training effect.

Most of us work out because we want to get faster or stronger or be able to go longer and harder at whatever we do, whether it's climbing up mountains or skiing down them. You want to test your limits and you don't want to slow down. Although you try to stay in shape, you encounter periods when your fitness declines because your training slacks off. Things get busy at work. You get a sore knee. Your treadmill breaks down. Whatever the reason, you periodically need to build yourself back up, and it's at those times that you return to the principles of overload and progression. So you start adding a few minutes to your stair machine workout, increase your long Sunday run, or add a second hard set to your daily swim workout. You start to push yourself.

Even fitness experts who once encouraged people to dally in the lower regions of their aerobic zone and convinced them that they would burn more fat walking moderately instead of running hard are starting to see the benefit of hard training. Pushing yourself even a little yields big gains on the fitness front. It makes your muscles get stronger and firmer, and, as we will explain in this chapter, it makes you a better fat-burning engine in many different ways.

How Your Body Produces Energy

To understand how to train and how the body reacts to training, a quick biology lesson might help. Molecules of adenosine triphosphate (ATP) provide the energy that triggers a muscle contraction. Covert Bailey, famous fitness scientist and author, likes to compare ATP to a common wooden kitchen match. The wooden shaft is the adenosine and the tip is the high-energy phosphorus that flames up and provides muscle cells

FAST-TWITCH AND SLOW-TWITCH MUSCLES

The muscles of the body are like the strings on a puppet. They are attached to our bones with fascia and tendons, and when they are activated by electrical impulses, they contract and pull the bones in a pattern that lets us run, ski, or swim. A skilled puppetmaster manipulates those strings with ease and grace, and so does a skilled athlete, whether she is a rock climber or ballerina.

The body is composed of both slow-twitch and fast-twitch muscles, and the percentage you have is based on heredity and not affected much by training. But the quality of work those muscles do and the percentage that will atrophy over time is strongly influenced by how (and how often) you put them to work.

We're talking here about voluntary muscles—the ones we can consciously control. These muscles comprise thousands of fibers, and each fiber is surrounded by a protective membrane and filled with sarcoplasm, a gelatin of protein filaments, mitochondria, and glycogen. You need an electron microscope to see this far down, but don't worry if you don't have one; even scientists aren't all that sure what happens inside the sarcoplasm to make a muscle quiver. The theory is that two types of proteins latch together like a couple of dancers in a Michael Jackson video and forcefully pull past each other. Thousands of filaments doing the same dance step simultaneously brings on the contraction you see when you flex your biceps.

A network of nerve cells that originate in the spinal cord coordinates these fiber contractions. These nerve-and-fiber teams are called motor units, and the size of a unit determines how fine the movement. For instance, the motor unit that controls the muscles in your voice box to produce those fine inflections of your voice is pretty small, maybe just two or three fibers. But when you are talking about the gastrocnemius muscle—that big one in your lower leg—the neurons are mobilizing something like 2,000 fibers into action.

Fibers are either fast-twitch or slow-twitch fibers, and the difference is in the size of the unit and its skill at different types of work. In slow-twitch units, a small nerve cell commands anywhere from 10

with the energy they need. ATP is produced in the mitochondria, the areas your high school biology teacher called "the powerhouse of the cells." Because the body can't store much ATP and uses up its supplies within a few seconds, we have to recycle the burned up matches constantly by

to 180 fibers. In fast-twitch units, a large neuron oversees 300–800 fibers at one time. Slow-twitch units have good aerobic endurance and because that little neuron is easy to fire up, they are usually the first to roll into action. Fast-twitch fibers can produce a great deal more force, but they tire easily.

When you start out on an easy run or a swim, you'll use primarily slow-twitch fibers. As you work into it, however, and need greater speed or power, more and more fast-twitch fibers are called into play. Most people have either 60 percent slow-twitch fibers and the rest fast twitch or 60 percent fast-twitch fibers and 40 percent slow. Those with predominantly slow-twitch fibers are better suited to endurance events and those with more fast-twitch fibers would do better at explosive endeavors such as sprints or high-jumping.

You can develop the strength and aerobic capacity of muscles but you can't develop more fast-twitch fibers than you were born with. The secret for most people is to improve the aerobic capacities of their slow-twitch fibers so

they can be used at greater and greater speeds before getting clogged with lactic acid.

Most anaerobic training, the kind that leaves you breathless, puts your fast-twitch muscles to work. That's a good thing for many of us because those are the muscle fibers we are more likely to lose as we get older. If we are actively recruiting fast-twitch muscle fibers, they are much less likely to atrophy.

It's a common misperception that slow-twitch muscle fibers do all the work at low speeds and that fast twitch takes care of the high speeds. The truth is that they help each other out. Most endurance training—long, slower distance training—is handled by the slow twitch, but when those muscles become fatigued, the fast-twitch muscles roll into action and keep you going (not for long, but you can squeeze out several more minutes this way). Similarly, sprint training is primarily handled by fast-twitch muscles. When they become fatigued, the slow-twitch muscles jump into action. Of course, at this point you're not sprinting anymore.

replacing those expended phosphorus molecules. The first place we turn to is phosphocreatine, itself a high-energy, phosphate-bearing molecule in our muscles, but that supply only lasts about 5 to 10 seconds. At this point, oxygen hasn't even arrived on the scene yet, so the body starts to burn up sugar—glycogen and glucose—in the muscle to recycle the ATP. Unfortunately, it's not long before lactic acid, a byproduct of glycolysis, starts seeping into the muscles. Ouch. Finally, after just a minute or two of exercise, oxygen is delivered by your elevated breathing and heart rate and the job of recycling ATP falls to the aerobic machinery, which breaks down fat, carbohydrate, and protein for energy. That's what we're talking about when we talk about burning energy or burning fat. You are really just breaking down fat and sugar to recycle ATP so you have energy in a form your muscles can use.

Fat is a much better source of energy than sugar. We have a lot more fat in our body than glucose, and each fatty acid molecule releases a lot more energy than a glucose molecule. To release that abundant energy, though, you need fat-burning enzymes, and people who don't exercise don't have many of them.

Another problem with fat is that it can be burned only in the presence of oxygen. When you are walking or jogging easily, you are getting plenty of oxygen in your blood and you can burn a fair amount of fat. Fat burning also requires a little bit of sugar burning because it takes a long time to get the energy out of fat, and sugar is needed to keep the fire going while you wait. When you start working harder, however, your body starts to rely increasingly on sugar, which can be converted into energy faster than fat and doesn't need any oxygen. The problem is that this fast-burning anaerobic (no oxygen) process produces lactic acid, which builds up and starts to sting and sends us huffing and puffing to the side of the road. That's what happened to those guys on the treadmill.

The availability of energy is the most important factor governing maximum speed, overall pace, and general endurance. The secret to effective training, then, is to convince your body to make more aerobic energy available at faster and faster rates. And that's not hard to do. When you start pushing the body harder than it's used to going, it reacts in a pretty miraculous way: Your factory is suddenly able to recycle a whole lot more kitchen matches. That's why elite runners can burn 10 calories of fat per minute while exercising, whereas unfit people burn about 2 calories a minute exercising. The value of burning fat, beyond the fact that it will melt away your love handles, is that you always have fat to burn.

But getting there requires that you work all three of your energy delivery systems: your aerobic system, the fat- and sugar-burning process that requires oxygen but lets you work for a long time; your anaerobic system, the kind that burns sugar, requires no oxygen, lasts only 7 minutes, and usually leaves you stinging with lactic acid; and your creatine phosphate system. Creatine phosphate is that stuff 100-meter sprinters rely on to hurtle down the track. It is readily available in your cells for quick ATP recycling, but it only lasts just 5 or 10 seconds. Energy systems are like muscles: Only the ones that are stressed will adapt, and concentrating your training on one system causes the others to suffer. For example, swimmers who train solely at high intensity find that their endurance suffers. And runners who subscribe to the LSD theory of running (long, slow distance) find that they never get any faster.

"Gentle, lactic-acid–avoiding exercise will eventually get you fit," says Covert Bailey. "But that's not the most up-to-date advice. Some intense exercise . . . interspersed in an aerobic workout raises fitness much more quickly."

How Muscles Respond to Exercise

It may be your muscles that get sore or sting from lactic acid, but exercise really is raising the ante for every part of your body. The liver is forced to produce glycogen more efficiently, and the pancreas adjusts the rate at which it releases insulin and glucose. The lungs increase their volume and learn to deliver more oxygen. The heart gets stronger and pumps more blood with each beat. Your circulatory system actually starts building new pathways—called capillaries—into the fibers of muscles that are calling out for oxygen, sugar, and fatty acids, thus making it easier to deliver more fuel and release heat. Endurance-trained swimmers have up to 50 percent more capillaries in their arm muscles than sedentary people do.

The muscle itself responds by building more and larger mitochondria, increasing its ability to replenish ATP stores. The leg muscles of a marathon runner, for instance, have three times the aerobic capacity of the legs of a sedentary person. That's a lot of hard-working, hungry mitochondria. The production of ATP in the mitochondria depends on oxidative enzymes, and the amount of oxidative enzymes also increases as you get fit, to anywhere from two to three times the number you'll find in someone who doesn't work out. The muscle also increases its supply of myoglobin, which acts as a storage compartment in the muscle for oxygen and allows the muscle to continue working aerobically when oxygen in the blood is running short.

In recent years researchers have noticed another adaptation to exercise: higher levels of fat in the muscle. It may seem odd that a fit person would have more fat in his or her muscle, but this fat is in the form of triglycerides, which break down into fatty acids, and in a fit person you'll find them right next to the mitochondria. Unfit people will find triglycerides in other places, including their hips, bellies, and thighs. Triglycerides float around in the bloodstream looking for a hungry muscle, like a waiter cruising a busy restaurant with a coffeepot, looking for somebody who wants a refill. If nobody wants him, the waiter takes a seat with the other triglycerides in your butt or your love handles.

And once fat is stored, it takes longer to mobilize it. When an unfit person starts to exercise and wants some of that fat to burn, it can take the body up to 30 minutes to release it and get it down to the mitochondria to do some work. People who exercise more often gain access to that fat a lot sooner, maybe in 15 minutes. A really fit person has immediate access. Not only does the body learn to release fatty acids faster, but it also has learned to store some droplets of fat right in the muscle fiber. After only eight weeks of endurance running, for instance, your muscle triglyceride content will be almost twice what it was before. And you'll have more fat-burning enzymes around to process it.

The result of all these adaptations—increased number of capillaries, more mitochondria, and more myoglobin—is that you can burn fat sooner, faster, and longer. That's why marathoner Alberto Salazar can run 5-minute miles in a marathon and still be drawing 70 to 80 percent of his energy from fat.

Exercise also encourages your body to do a better job of storing and replenishing glycogen. When endurance athletes cut back on their training and eat a diet rich in carbohydrates, their muscle glycogen levels increase to twice the levels of sedentary people. That's not a result of gluttony; it's an adaptation to training.

Glycogen is formed from a string of glucose (blood sugar) molecules, and any increase in the storage of it is key because you still need to burn a little sugar to burn fat, and glycogen is in short supply in the body. You can burn up your glycogen stores fairly quickly if you are working so hard that your body can't use fat fast enough to recycle the ATP. But even if you are working more slowly and getting only 20 percent of your energy from glycogen, it will eventually run out. That's why ultramarathoners and cyclists in the Tour de France eat so much during their events; they don't want to run out of blood sugar.

EXERCISE TEACHES YOUR BODY TO BURN FAT SOONER, FASTER, AND LONGER.

The catch is that your body can only replenish its glycogen stores so fast. For instance, unfit people can restore it at a rate of only 5 percent an hour. But training can get that rate up to 10 percent an hour.

One of the side benefits of getting in good shape is that your body will continue to burn fat after you've stopped exercising. After a workout, your body sets to work replenishing its glycogen stores. It needs ATP to do this. That means it needs energy. So it burns fat. That's why your heart rate usually remains elevated after you've quit exercising and why you might feel a rush of heat an hour or so after working out. This period of restoration also explains why it is important to eat within 2 hours after exercise. It's called the glycogen window, and research has shown that glycogen is replaced 50 percent faster in athletes who eat between 15 and 30 minutes after they finish exercise. The best thing to eat? Some athletes save their bars, gels, cookies, and sports drinks for the minute they get off the trail, and that's good because simple sugars enter the bloodstream and the muscle much faster than complex carbohydrates.

The Fundamentals of Training

So how do you convince your body to make all these changes? As we said earlier, a good training program is one in which you push both your aerobic system (endurance) and your anaerobic system (speed). Everybody knows what endurance training is: It's long, slower distance training at anywhere from 50 to 75 percent of your MHR. So let's talk about anaerobic training first because that's the one that usually scares people the most and makes them stop training altogether.

Anaerobic training is simply training at a speed or effort level that is just beyond your body's aerobic comfort zone. It is this kind of training that forces some of the adaptations in the body that we've already talked about. When your body, accustomed to running at an aerobic pace that

LACTIC ACID: FEEL THE BURN

For years, the standard used to gauge an athlete's fitness was VO_2 max, which is the maximum amount of oxygen a person can consume during 1 minute of hard exercise. Scientists believed that any athlete with a chart-busting VO_2 max would outperform anyone with a more pedestrian score.

But that isn't always the case. Olympic runners Frank Shorter and Derek Clayton had modest VO_2 max scores and were beating athletes with higher readings. Why? Because Shorter and Clayton had higher lactate thresholds; they had trained themselves to run aerobically at very high speeds and as a result were using a greater percentage of their VO_2 max before their bodies started burning sugar and accumulating debilitating

amounts of lactic acid.

VO_2 max is hereditary and can be improved only modestly through training, but your lactic threshold can be greatly improved by training. A swimmer with a VO_2 max of 60 milliliters of oxygen per minute per kilogram of body weight who can swim at 92 percent of her maximum before reaching her lactate threshold will perform better than a swimmer with a VO_2 max of 65 who reaches only 75 percent of her maximum. VO_2 max is a measure of your potential, but lactate threshold is a measure of your fitness.

Lactic acid is being produced long before we feel it. Right after it's produced, lactic acid splits into hydrogen ions and lactate. The hydrogen ions are dealt with by the body's bicarbonate buffering sys-

allows it to burn a lot of fat, is suddenly pushed to the point where it is burning more sugar and accumulating lactic acid, it responds by improving blood flow, increasing its supply of fat-burning enzymes, and triggering the release of fatty acids sooner. As these adaptations take place, you slowly get used to running at that faster pace and it becomes an aerobic pace for you. Then you have to step it up again. This type of training is called lactate threshold because you are training at a level where you are very close to flooding your body with lactic acid.

Another goal of anaerobic training is to teach you to better tolerate lactic acid. With this kind of training, you are going fast enough to produce a good supply of lactic acid. You really feel the burn. It may sting a little, but there is a lot of value in this type of training.

tem, which binds the ions to bicarbonate to form carbonic acid that then splits into carbon dioxide and water, which the body can get rid of pretty easily. The lactate is actually used as a fuel source by nonworking muscles and the heart and liver, both of which reform the lactate into glucose. You reach your lactic threshold when you can't recycle the lactic acid fast enough.

How do you know you are there? If you are running or cycling, gradually speed up over a 10-minute period to a point where your legs feel like rubber and your breathing increases in a pronounced way. If you were breathing every third step and suddenly you are breathing every other step, you are probably at your lactate threshold. If you're unfit, you are probably at 50 or 60 percent of your MHR;

fit people can reach 90 percent before they are on the verge of going anaerobic.

The secret to improving your ability to neutralize lactic acid is to work out for a sustained period (20–30 minutes) just at or below your lactic threshold. You can either keep up the effort for a sustained period or break it up into long intervals with short recovery periods. If you do 10 to 20 percent of your total weekly workload at your lactate threshold, you'll see big improvements in just six to nine workouts. Say you do a 3-mile run in 19 minutes and your heart rate is at 160 beats per minute. After several weeks, your time for that 3-mile run should drop even though you keep your heart rate at 160 beats per minute. You're on your way to becoming the next Frank Shorter.

You are actually teaching the body to produce more lactic acid, and the advantage of this is that you learn to generate more energy from this source before you get fatigued. Unlike endurance training, where you work out easily for a long time with very short rest breaks, sprint training is working out very hard for a short period with long rest breaks. And by "rest" we mean recovery periods. This usually involves slow, easy exercise that allows the lactic acid produced by all that hard-core sugar burning to seep into your slow-twitch and nonworking muscles and get consumed aerobically. Swimmers, for instance, swim an easy 200 after a set of sprints. Runners who are doing 400-meter repeats on the track jog 400 meters between their hard runs.

- DEVELOP A PLAN.

- ALTERNATE EASY AND HARD WORKOUTS.

- FIND A TRAINING PARTNER.

This kind of training is called lactate tolerance, and it improves the muscle's buffering capacity, or its ability to withstand the fatigue that comes with a lactic acid invasion. Researchers have found that after only eight weeks of sprint training, a muscle's buffering capacity will increase up to 50 percent. Another advantage of lactate tolerance training is that you teach yourself to withstand the pain better, allowing you to stay at that pace longer than before. This is a psychological adaptation, and you can't really measure it. Some people seem to handle the pain better than others.

Does training at these levels seem out of the question for you? It doesn't have to be. Even if you are a casual exerciser—an avid hiker, for instance, or maybe an occasional jogger—it's important to realize that all you are doing by weaving some hard training into your repertoire is forcing more beneficial adaptations from your body. You are already demanding changes of your body, and there is nothing particularly painful or pretentious about demanding even more. If you are a walker, try throwing in some jogging. If you are a steady lap swimmer, try including a set of sprints in your workout. You might be surprised at the additional speed and strength—not to mention the elevated sense of well-being—that more intense exercise will bring you.

That said, the best distances for lactate tolerance training are those that can be covered in 45 seconds to 2 minutes. For swimmers, that usually means any distance between 75 and 200 yards or meters and for runners that means anywhere from 300 to 800 meters. The rest period is however long it takes to dissipate the lactic acid buildup (sometimes up to 5 minutes). You go all out in these sprints—maximum speed—but you only need to do a handful before your muscles give out.

One thing that confuses people is the term *interval training*. This means taking a certain distance and chopping it up into smaller portions. You run or swim or ski these intervals at a predetermined pace with a predetermined rest period. Intervals can be done at lactate tolerance pace—a sprint—but you can also do endurance training in an interval format. Distance swimmers often do this. If you are doing an endurance workout this way, the key is to maintain your pace and to take only very short rests.

The Ideal Training Program

Some older athletes maintain the same volume of training as they age, and others increase the volume. But many slowly decrease the intensity of their workouts. The experts aren't sure why, but they think it's a reflection of changing interests. It's easier for jobs and other obligations to interfere as you get older, and some athletes lose interest in the competitions that usually inspire them to train hard. Whatever the reason, it doesn't make sense from a physiological standpoint because studies have shown that older athletes can continue to handle hard workouts. Some argue that these kinds of workouts become increasingly important as an athlete tries to maintain strength and speed with age. Although many older athletes worry more about injuries caused by hard training than they used to and some contend that they don't recover as quickly from hard training as they once did, it's still important to find the right balance in your training. Keep your hard lactate threshold and tolerance workouts, but make sure you follow them with days of rest or easy training. Most of us tend to train too hard on our easy days, which affects the quality of our hard days. So find the right balance and stick to it.

Whether you are a fitness swimmer or runner or an avid racer, some basic principles apply to all training programs. The key is to develop long-range goals. Look past next week's workouts or even this summer's exercise plan. The biggest mistake athletes make is adding too much work too quickly and getting injured or sick. This is particularly true of athletes approaching their fiftieth birthday. They think at fifty they will begin the quick slide into senior citizenship and that this is their last chance to go really fast. Don't fall into that trap. And don't fall into the trap of thinking that exercise has to be painful and tedious. What it should be, more than anything else, is fun. If you don't enjoy it, you won't stay with it.

We'll go into more detail about training in later chapters on the in-

CROSS-TRAINING: WHEN OPPOSING MUSCLES WORK TOGETHER

Cross-training—any training program designed to work different muscle groups in different ways—is a great way to prevent injuries and to recover from them. Up to 70 percent of runners are injured badly enough each year that they cannot train. For these people, who will lose nearly 20 percent of their aerobic capacity after just six weeks of inactivity (that's like aging twenty years), cross-training is the best way to keep from losing what they've worked so hard to build.

Injured runners can turn to a number of alternatives. One of the better ones is cycling, which doesn't involve the pounding that running does and works the quadriceps and lateral upper leg muscles, which are often weak in runners and responsible for knee pain and imbalance injuries in the groin area. Stair machines can also help your running. In one study,

subjects worked out on stair climbers 30–45 minutes a day, 4 days a week for nine weeks. They worked at anywhere from 70 to 90 percent of their MHRs. The result? Their times for a 1.5-mile run improved by a minute.

Then there is water running. Some argue that water running—running in place in the deep end of the pool—isn't so much cross-training as it is supplemental training because you're using the same motions. But water is far denser than air, and this makes it a different exercise. Running in the water works the entire body, including the arms and the chest, and there is resistance against the leg muscles in all phases of the motion, including the recovery. In one study, athletes who trained for six weeks in the water improved their times for a 2-mile run.

Swimming works upper-body areas

dividual sports, but for now, here are the principles for building a good training program in any sport:

- **Develop a plan for the entire year.** If you want to do a race or special undertaking, such as climbing Mount Whitney, build up to it and plan your year around the month or two when you want to be in top form. That means you'll have a period of two to three months where you are doing mostly basic endurance training. Swimmers and cross-country skiers use this time to work on their

neglected by running, cycling, and walking. That makes it a good complement. Many triathletes feel swimming improves their flexibility and makes them better runners. One thing to keep in mind if you water run or swim is that your heart rate will be about 10 beats less than when you're on land exercising.

Perhaps the greatest benefit of cross-training is that it keeps your workouts fresh. It's easier to do tough back-to-back workouts; you can run on Wednesday, swim on Thursday, and still have fresh legs for a run on Friday.

And cross-training is a good way to achieve better overall fitness. Fitness guidelines, which once addressed only aerobic exercise, now recommend adding some strength training to your workouts. That usually means working on your upper body, and such cross-training sports as cross-country skiing and swimming do just that. So if your primary exercise is running, hiking, or cycling, you should consider adding another sport or taking up weightlifting to improve your overall fitness.

What follows are some major sports and what the experts feel are complementary cross-training sports:

- Running: Cycling, stairs, water running, and cross-country skiing
- Swimming: Cross-country skiing (although even that sport won't improve a highly technical activity like swimming)
- Cross-country skiing: Running, rock climbing, in-line skating, cycling
- Cycling: Weight training, cross-country skiing, in-line or speed skating, running
- Rowing: Cross-country skiing, weight training, swimming

technique. This period is followed by increasingly intense workouts in which you raise your aerobic and anaerobic capacities. You are still doing a lot of basic endurance training but an increasing amount of your endurance training is in the intense category—say 70 to 90 percent of your MHR. Finally, you add some sharpening training, in which you focus more and more on race-pace training. You'll do more anaerobic training and sprinting and less basic endurance. You are now in your race season. When the season is over, relax and back off; no one can stay in top shape all year.

- **Plan your training week around your tough workouts.** Swimmers can do only two tough sets back to back before they must revert to easy endurance swims while their bodies restore all that spent glycogen. Runners typically shoot for 3 tough days: a speed session on the track or grass, a tempo run in which they go hard for an extended period at near race pace, and a long run that is at an easy pace but stresses the body's energy supply. Cross-country skiers plan their weeks around two hard interval sessions with repeats of 3 to 8 minutes.

- **Remember to alternate hard and easy.** Although some elite athletes train hard 2 days in a row (ultramarathoners do this when they follow their 40-mile Saturday run with a 20- or 30-mile Sunday jaunt in preparation for 100-mile races), most have learned to follow a tough day with an easy day. Using the hard–easy system has a couple of advantages: It gives your body time to heal itself and restore lost energy, and it gives you a mental break from training. When your hard day comes, you are more eager for it. And when that workout is over and lactic acid is dripping from your pores, you can look forward to the next day's easy workout. There are variations of the hard–easy principle. Ultrarunners who do back-to-back hard days usually take it easy for 2 or 3 days after. And some athletes take 2 easy days after a hard lactate tolerance or lactate threshold workout. Some guidelines: Take 2 days after any ski, run, or bike ride that's more than 30 percent of your weekly mileage. Also, make sure on your easy days to work those tired muscles just a little bit; that stimulates them to heal faster.

And don't increase your mileage by adding miles to your easy day; add them to your hard days.

- **Have some variety.** Change pools once in a while. Run with some different people. Get off the groomed ski trails and go backcountry occasionally. Train with different people now and then. Go on an adventure workout, where you ride, climb, or paddle somewhere you've never been.

- **Make it fun for the whole family.** Find ways to work out with your kids. When they are babies, take them with you in a baby jogger. Tow them around in a bike trailer or a ski sled. When they get older, let them ride along with you on their bikes while you run or roller ski. Some open-water swimmers tow their kids on boogie boards while they freestyle across a lake. Now that's resistance training.

INVOLVE THE WHOLE FAMILY.

- **Get a training partner.** They get you out on days you might stay in, they push you to greater heights, and they stop and walk with you when you just can't push yourself anymore. They also provide great training options. You can do pursuit workouts, where you alternate chasing down your partner. If you have a choice, pick a partner who is a little faster than you. This will help you improve and probably keep him or her from overtraining.

- **Keep a training log.** For some people, these are dangerous things. They become slaves to them and they work out more than they should just so they can put up big numbers. But if you have a training program and a log to record your efforts, you are less likely to skip a day. You'll know when it's time to boost your intensity level, and when it comes time to race you will have written proof that you have done the preparation. This will keep you from second-guessing yourself before a race, worrying about whether you've trained hard enough.

- **Learn what is hard and what is easy for you.** The best way is to go by your heart rate and your percentage of total weekly mileage (workload). For instance, you can be running easy (at only 60 to 70 percent of your MHR) but it's a hard day if you do more than 20 percent of your weekly mileage that day. If you're doing a speed workout near or at your MHR, don't do more than 10 percent of your total weekly mileage.

- **Keep in mind that there are limits.** Any athlete who works hard enough will eventually reach his or her maximum levels. Should this discourage you? No! When your physiological system is tapped out, look for ways to become more efficient. Get a coach to help with your swimming stroke or your skating technique. Learn more about waxing your skis to make them faster. Do some cross-training. Try a new sport altogether. You may find that swimming wasn't the best sport for you, that you are a natural born cross-country skier.

CHAPTER 4

HOW MUCH EXERCISE IS ENOUGH?

Bjorn Daehlie, the legendary Norwegian cross-country skier, is known for his grueling training schedule. He works out up to 8 hours a day, and over the course of a year his training log might show he's trained more than 1,000 hours.

Even if you had the time, chances are you wouldn't train that much. But you've probably asked yourself at one time or another whether you're training hard enough or long enough to achieve your goals. If you're walking 2 miles a day, should you start running? If you're running 20 miles a week, will 30 make you stronger or faster?

The truth is, these questions are almost impossible to answer.

We do know that some exercise is better than none and that more vigorous exercise reaps vastly greater benefits than moderate exercise. But how hard should you go? How far? How often? Nobody knows. Kenneth Cooper, the father of aerobics who once advocated such excessive training as marathon running, now says running more than 30 miles a week releases free radicals in your body that can destroy healthy tissues. Other fitness experts who once advised people to walk if they wanted to burn fat now tell people they should do wind sprints along with their endurance training.

Confused? No wonder.

What Should I Do to Get Started?

Just start walking. Walk every day for at least 2 miles and do it like you mean it. Walk briskly, swinging your arms, and don't stop until you are through. What's more, time yourself. Every once in a while, try to get a little faster. When you start seeing yourself getting faster, add some distance and walk longer. When you feel up to it, get a pair of good running shoes and start jogging short stretches of your walk.

Although the American College of Sports Medicine (ACSM) and the Center for Disease Control claim you get almost the same benefit from walking three times a day for 10 minutes each time as you can from one continuous 30-minute walk, new studies being done at Cooper's Institute of Aerobics Research in Dallas don't bear that out. There, researchers are comparing people who do structured, continuous, health-club–style workouts with those who are accumulating their 30 minutes. Those who are accumulating their workouts are getting the same benefits, such as higher HDL levels (the "good" cholesterol), less body fat, and lower blood pressure, but they are acquiring these benefits at half the rate of those doing continuous exercise every day.

If you are not fit, walking will burn more fat than running. That's because running, for you, would be anaerobic, and as we learned in the last chapter, anaerobic exercise burns sugar for energy. But it takes a long time to burn fat when you're walking, and your body will never learn to burn fat at faster speeds unless you overload it and stress it sometimes. Stressing it with short stretches of jogging will convince your body to start delivering fat to running muscles, and in time you will start burning fat while you're jogging. When you start getting into this kind of shape, not only will you burn more fat when you exercise, but you'll start burning it sooner.

There are other benefits to more vigorous exercise. In the Harvard Alumni Health Study, mortality rates among men who burned 3,500 calories per week—that's a good, hard, half-hour run every day—were about half those of the men who burned just 500 calories a week. Another study in the January 1998 issue of *Archives of Internal Medicine* found that men who ran 40 miles or more each week had a 30 percent lower risk of coronary heart disease than those who ran 10 miles a week.

Be forewarned: Beginning joggers have more foot, leg, and knee

MODERATE AND INTENSE LEVELS OF EXERCISE

Kenneth Cooper recommends these guidelines for moderate and vigorous exercise:

Moderate Levels of Exercise

- Walk 2 miles in less than 30 minutes three times a week.
- Walk 2 miles in less than 40 minutes four times a week.
- Walk 2 miles in less than 45 minutes five times a week.

Vigorous Levels of Exercise

- Run 2 miles in less than 20 minutes four times a week.
- Walk 3 miles in less than 45 minutes five times a week.
- Take four 45-minute aerobics classes each week.

injuries when they are running more than 3 days a week for more than 30 minutes each time. And women tend to have more orthopedic injuries than men: twice as many when they are younger and four times as many when they get older. Scientists aren't sure why women get injured so much more than men the same age, but one reason could be that they have less muscle mass in their lower extremities. To avoid injury, stretch carefully before and after exercise, and back off from the intensity of your workout if you start to feel any pain in your joints.

The American College of Sports Medicine's aerobic guidelines still call for 20–60 minutes of aerobic training 3–5 days a week at 60 to 90 percent of your MHR. For most people, that's considerably more demanding than a brisk 2-mile walk. But if you stay within that 60 to 90 percent MHR range—moderate to high intensity—you can significantly cut your risk of such problems as diabetes, coronary disease, colon cancer, and osteoporosis. Easy walking won't do much more than lower your blood pressure.

Priming the Pump: Training with Heart Rate

Although many athletes determine their training loads by sheer mileage, the smart ones train according to time and effort level. They know that not all 4-mile runs are the same. Some 4-milers on a flat grassy area are recovery runs. A 4-miler on a rocky trail that gains 2,000 feet in elevation is a much harder session that may warrant a day off to recover.

Many athletes train according to feel or by a perceived effort level, but heart rate monitoring takes a lot of the guesswork out of your training and prevents you from training too hard or too casually. Every person has a maximum heart rate, and working out at different percentages of that rate puts different demands on the body and results in different adaptations that make you stronger and more resilient.

Working out at 60 to 70 percent of your MHR teaches your heart to pump more blood more efficiently, increases blood flow and enzymes in the muscle, builds muscle endurance, and enhances your body's ability to burn fat as a fuel. You should stay in this zone for easy recovery workouts and for your long, endurance-building workouts.

Working out at around 90 percent of your MHR improves your body's ability to burn fat at high effort levels—something you'll need to improve your speed over longer distances. It's called lactate threshold training because it's the point where you are toying with a serious invasion of lactic acid brought on by burning too much sugar and not enough fat for energy. Training above 90 percent is called lactate tolerance training because you are encouraging your body to burn up sugar so you can get it accustomed to the sting of lactic acid, something you're bound to encounter at some point in a race or a steep hill.

Finding the right mix of both these types of workouts is the secret to good fitness in any sport.

Your heart rate is also a bellwether for a great many other things. A resting heart rate that declines over time is a good sign that you're getting more fit. But if you're finding that your resting heart rate, taken first thing in the morning before you get up, is increasing, it may be a sign of illness or overtraining.

HEART RATE MONITORING CAN PREVENT YOU FROM TRAINING TOO HARD OR TOO CASUALLY.

You can also use your heart rate to measure your progress. Say you do a 3-mile run in 21 minutes at 160 beats per minute at the beginning of your training program. After a couple of months of training, your heart rate for the same distance and pace should be down to 145 beats per minute, indicating that you're in better shape and need to pick up the pace if you want to continue to improve.

Your heart lets you know not only whether you are working out hard enough, but also whether you're working out too hard. For instance, many runners like to do a tempo run once a week in which they run at their lactate thresholds for 20–30 minutes. They know from experience that the threshold is at 87 to 92 percent of their MHRs. Checking their heart rate along the way will let them know when they have reached that level. Going too hard leaves them gasping; instead of training your body to more efficiently remove lactate from your blood and burn fat at higher speeds, you'll be training your body to produce even more lactic acid—not the goal of this particular workout. It's also a good idea to monitor your heart on the easy days that follow a good tempo run; training too hard on a recovery day doesn't give your body the chance to refuel and do the repair work it needs and won't leave you fresh enough to take on another hard session in the next day or two.

By far the best way to keep track of your heart rate is with a monitor, which consists of a transmitter strapped around your chest and a receiver worn like a watch. Some models have headphones that relay information. You can get a basic unit for under $100, though there are more expensive systems that track your heart rate over time and interface with a computer to track your heart rate levels over time. Many of them have an annoying little beeping feature that goes off if your heart rate drops below a certain level or goes above a preset rate. There are even some treadmills that can be programmed to automatically adjust the speed and incline to keep you within a certain heart-rate zone. The advantage of a monitor is that you can check your heart rate during exercise. You don't have to stop and take your pulse—a method that is often off by as much as 20 beats per minute.

A BETTER WAY OF MEASURING YOUR HEART RATE

When serious athletes start using heart rate monitors and following training programs that require them to run at 60 or 70 percent of their MHRs, many have the same reaction: It doesn't feel hard enough.

Consider a forty-two-year-old runner who has an MHR of 180 beats per minute. If he runs at 60 percent of his maximum (180 x 0.60), his heart rate will only be 108 beats per minute. If he runs at 70 percent, his heart rate will be 126. At that rate, his running pace is extremely slow and he won't feel like he's working hard enough.

For that and other reasons, many athletes determine their training levels by using something called the heart rate reserve (HRR) method. Many feel this is the best way to prescribe exercise intensity because it takes into account your net heart rate, or how much your heart rate increases above resting values. For many athletes, exercise intensities make more sense when they are calculated as a percentage of HRR.

To calculate HRR, you need to know your MHR and your resting heart rate (RHR). Measure your MHR with a self-administered test on a track or pool or cycling route by thoroughly warming up and then methodically increasing your pace until you are going all-out for a sustained period (several minutes) and your heart rate has leveled off. Measure your RHR first thing in the morning before

Finding Your Maximum Heart Rate

The secret to effective heart-rate training is knowing your MHR. This is pretty much determined by your genes, and is one of the few things that declines with age no matter how hard you exercise.

There are several ways to estimate your MHR. The most common formula is 220 minus your age. This is a good starting point for people just starting a fitness program, but it's accurate for only about a third of the people who use it. If you're a veteran athlete, a better equation is 205 minus half your age, which will give you a higher reading but is likely to be more accurate.

The most reliable measure is to get a stress test on a treadmill. You go to a lab, get hooked up to a monitor, and then submit yourself to the resident sadist at the controls. A stress test starts slowly—a pace about 4 minutes a mile below your best effort—but very slowly and

getting out of bed (do this for several mornings and take the average).

To get your training heart rate (THR), subtract your RHR from your MHR and multiply that figure by the percentage you want to train at. Then add the RHR back in to arrive at the heart rate you want to train at.

The formula looks like this: THR = [(MHR - RHR) x intensity percentage] + RHR.

So let's say the forty-two-year-old runner has a resting heart rate of 43. To get a 60 percent training heart rate you would subtract 43 from 180 and get 137. Then you would multiply that by 0.60 and get 82.2. When you add back the 43 resting heart rate, you get 125.2 as his

training heart rate for training at 60 percent effort. That feels more like it. His heart rate at 70 percent is 138–139.

The differences between HRR and regular heart rate training become less noticeable as the percentages increase. A 90 percent HRR training level is 166, for instance, and 162 if you just take a percentage of your MHR.

Using a percentage of your HRR will give you a better idea of how much oxygen you are consuming and it allows you to adjust for changes in your RHR. The math might be too demanding for people in oxygen debt, so figure your percentages ahead of time, jot them down on a small scrap of paper, and tape it to your watchband so you can refer to it.

methodically gets tougher. You keep going until your heart rate levels off and the lab tech takes pity on you.

You can replicate this test on your own at a track and get similar results. You start out running each lap at about a minute slower than what you think your pace would be for a fast 2-mile run, and you whittle 15 seconds off each lap until you are at that race pace. You stay at that pace for two laps and then you crank it up even more. On the last two laps, you are running full throttle and checking your heart rate every 100 meters. When it reaches its peak and won't go any higher, you can stop, pick up the vital organs that have spilled all over the track, and go home knowing that you can now develop some pacing guidelines that will make you extremely fit.

Cyclists, skiers, and swimmers can perform similar tests, the goal being to work steadily into a strong race pace and then into an all-out effort. It's important that you work into it—jumping into a maximum pace too quickly won't give you're an accurate measure. It's also important to know that your MHR is not the same for all sports, even if you're in top shape for them. For instance, your MHR in swimming will be 10–13 beats per minute slower because your body is horizontal, the water pressure helps push the blood back to the heart, and the water has a cooling effect. This doesn't mean that if you swim you don't have to work out as hard. It just means that you shouldn't be discouraged when you swim a hard set of 100s and notice that your heart rate is lower than expected.

Your MHR also tends to be lower when you're cycling. And your heart rate will vary according to what cycling position you are in. If your body is horizontal to the ground, your hands on the drops of your road bike, your heart rate will be lower than when you are sitting upright.

What Happens When You Overdo It

There is a fine line between overloading—the process of systematically increasing your workload so you can get faster or stronger—and overtraining, a mysterious malady that is, in many ways, the purgatory of endurance athletes.

If your idea of hell is a place where everything is upside down, illogical, and relentlessly confounding, then overtraining fits in like fire and wailing souls. When you've crossed the line from smart training to overtraining, nothing is as it seems.

You are dog-tired, yet you can't sleep. You need to eat, but you're not hungry. The training runs that once triggered that sweet release of goodwill and satisfaction (endorphins) now leave you in a black mood. The bones that once got stronger now get weaker, and the very muscles you are training aren't getting stronger and larger, they are getting weaker and smaller. The very same habits that once made you resistant to disease now make you more susceptible.

What's worse is that you respond to all this bad news by doing the worst thing you could do: You train harder.

Overtraining is not as uncommon as you might think. According to the National Institutes of Health, 60 to 64 percent of all elite long-distance runners in this country will go stale at some point in their careers and suffer from overtraining. Staleness will bother up to 30 percent of all serious recreational athletes, and a milder form of overtraining can strike many others who are training for fitness.

What causes overtraining? Scientists are still sorting out the physical reasons for it. It's probably related to a low energy supply to the muscles, a situation that forces the body to discourage more exercise until stores can be replenished. Some researchers have also blamed free radicals—groups of atoms that accumulate during endurance training and can damage DNA and muscle cells. When you start accumulating a lot of free radicals, you may start damaging tissue faster than you can repair it, and your power, speed, and endurance decline.

There is also evidence that people can push themselves to illness. People who run more than 60 miles a week are twice as likely to get sick as those running 20. And when researchers studied a group of marathoners, they found that of those who trained for the 26.2-mile race but did not run the actual race, only 2 percent got sick. Of those who ran the race, 13 percent got sick. The implication is that those who got sick crossed some kind of threshold in which energy intended for their immune systems was sidetracked to their exercise systems. They went too far.

The risks of overtraining are particularly severe for women, who can suffer from early osteoporosis, amenorrhea, and infertility if they train extremely hard and don't give their bodies the fuel they need to repair the damage and restock for the next workout. Female athletes also have a greater risk of anemia. Anemia is caused by a drop in red blood cells and a corresponding drop in blood hemoglobin, which delivers oxygen to your muscles. Less hemoglobin means less oxygen, and that means less speed and endurance. The body is pretty good at rebuilding hemoglobin—those molecules are constantly disintegrating and being built back up—but it needs iron to do it, and hard training often diminishes the amount of iron available in your body to rebuild hemoglobin. When that happens, you notice that your heart rate is faster than it should be at easy training levels and that you produce more lactic acid than you normally would at higher rates of training.

HEART RATE TIPS

Here are some other things to keep in mind when measuring your heart rate:

- Women's MHR is typically lower than men's but their heart rates are likely to be higher for the same effort level as men. And their hearts don't recover as quickly.

- High altitude will cause your heart rate to go up until your body reacts by creating more oxygen-carrying red blood cells. That's why a lot of world-class athletes train at high altitudes; all those extra red blood cells make them feel tireless when they run at sea level.

- Your heart rate will increase when it's cold and when it's hot. In one case the body is trying to maintain its core temperature. In the other, it's sending blood to the skin to try and keep the body cool. Either way, it may appear that you are working out harder than you are. That's why you tend to run more slowly in 95-degree heat.

- Don't be surprised by cardiac drift. If you are doing a long workout at a steady rate of intensity, your heart rate will slowly increase, even though you aren't pushing yourself any harder. This is probably the result of declining plasma volume due to sweating. Stay hydrated to offset the effect.

Can women handle the same training load as men? In most cases, yes. How much most of us train is determined pretty much by how much time we've got anyway. At the elite level, coaches in some sports believe women perform best when their training volume is 10 to 15 percent less than the level done by elite male athletes. Any more than that, and the women often become overtrained. The difference, some experts say, is that men have higher average testosterone levels and can grow and repair tissues faster than women.

Diagnosing and Treating Overtraining Problems

How do you tell if you're overtrained? Scientists have taken a whack at that, too, but with mixed results. One telltale factor is low levels of the amino acid glutamine. Low levels of glutamine result in poor cell reproduction and, consequently, a poor defense against bacteria and viruses. Researchers studying overtrained athletes have also found high levels of cortisol, a hormone responsible for the maintenance of normal blood glucose and free fatty acids, the stuff we use to recycle ATP during exercise. Scientists have also noticed that overtrained athletes have an elevated level of creatine kinase, an enzyme in muscles associated with ATP recycling. It's normally very high in muscles that have been damaged, but it's also been found in high levels in overtrained athletes who aren't feeling any pain in their muscles.

Because you probably don't have blood-testing facilities at your house, there are other ways to tell whether you're getting overtrained. Besides the sleeplessness, irritability, more frequent colds, and a drop in performance, you'll also notice that your resting heart rate is getting higher. Researchers say anywhere from 6 to 10 beats per minute higher is a good sign you're overtraining. If you wear a heart rate monitor during exercise, you'll notice that your rate will be unusually high for easy or moderate exercise. One study found a cross-country runner whose heart rate was 18 percent higher than it normally was for a moderate run. You may also notice that it takes longer for your elevated heart rate to return to normal after you finish exercising. One sure-fire clue for swimmers is when their race-pace stroke rate increases and their times do not improve.

Older athletes whose bodies don't repair themselves as quickly as they once did also have to beware of overtraining. We've all seen older runners—say in their sixties or seventies—who are good runners and extremely healthy but appear to be somewhat emaciated. Their legs are strong, but their upper bodies, for instance, look almost withered. These are people who aren't giving their bodies enough time to replenish their glycogen stores before their next workout. When they set off on another run and the call goes out from the muscles for some glycogen to burn, their liver reroutes some amino acids intended for rebuilding muscles and sends it down for use in aerobic metabolism. The result is that non-working muscles—such as those in the neck, shoulders, chest, and arms—get shortchanged. This can also happen in much younger athletes.

When this happens, the best thing to do is to back way off for any-where from 3 days to a week. Light, easy-pace training at greatly reduced distances might help you, but complete rest will never hurt. If you're not seeing improvement after a week off from heavy work, you may have to take more elaborate steps. Take a week off completely—no training whatsoever—and when you return, do only light to moderate training. Take some time to deal with some of the other things that might be both-ering you—work, home, whatever it is. You should also be increasing your carbohydrate intake. Some athletes get massages, and coaches in Australia have had some success putting athletes in isolation tanks for complete relaxation.

More and more endurance sport coaches are subscribing to the free-radical theory and urging their athletes to supplement their di-ets with vitamins C and E and beta-carotene. How much? Swimmers in heavy training take 400–1,000 mg of vitamin C a day, 400–1,000 mg of vitamin E and 5,000–8,000 IU of beta-carotene.

One of the terrible truths about training and exercise is that the better you get, the harder you have to work to achieve more. A beginning athlete might invest 100 hours of training in one season and see a 20 percent improvement in her performance. The next year it might be 200 hours for a 10 percent improvement, then 300 hours for 5 percent. As she approaches the peak of her career, she might be putting in 1,000 hours—Bjorn Daehlie levels of training—to gain a single percentage point. You are investing in a business with diminishing returns, but sometimes that percentage point you gain is the difference between a gold medal and a silver medal.

The bottom line is that you have to approach training cautiously: Build slowly and monitor your progress. If your performance starts to decline, you may have gone too far. If it levels off, you may need to go further. Finding the right training level is the science of finding the right amount of volume and intensity, and this requires patience and an understanding of how much stress to put on your body. It's also important to keep in mind that there is a limit for everyone—a point where no matter how much work you do, you can't get any faster or stronger. Of course, not too many people have reached that limit and those who do probably wouldn't believe it anyway.

Weight Training for Older Athletes

Weight training is particularly important as you get older and start losing muscle. One estimate claims the average man will lose 15 pounds of muscle by age fifty if he does no exercise at all. That muscle loss, called sarcopenia, starts at age thirty-five or younger and even vigorous aerobic exercise can't hold it off. A long-term study at Ball State University in Indiana found that a group of very fit runners over sixty years old lost 7 pounds of muscle mass after their fortieth birthdays despite maintaining an ongoing and intense aerobic schedule. Running just isn't enough.

The American College of Sports Medicine recommends strength training 2–3 days a week, doing 8 to 10 exercises that use all the major muscle groups in the body—including the arms, shoulders, chest, back, abdominals, hips, and legs. Pick a weight you can lift 8 but no more than 12 times. The American College of Sports Medicine recommends doing that many repetitions at least once. You can use either free weights or weight machines.

Others recommend more repetitions with less weight. For instance, advisors for Team Oregon, a running club, recommend starting with two or three circuits of 10 reps and building up to five to seven circuits of 20–30 reps. These exercises are done quickly and should take no more than 30–40 minutes. The runners who do these workouts don't take their muscles to exhaustion like most weightlifters; they prefer to develop their muscles' aerobic capacities.

Although most experts recommend two or three weightlifting workouts a week, one study shows that people can make significant improvements in their muscle strength and tone by lifting weights only twice a week for 20–30 minutes with no warmup.

WEIGHT TRAINING IS INDISPENSABLE FOR THE OLDER ATHLETE.

A couple of things to keep in mind:

- Never use more weight than you can lift correctly.
- Take a class or get help from a trainer if you've never lifted before.
- Use the mirrors in your gym to practice correct form.
- Never snap your knees or elbows; press the weight slowly, stopping before completely extending the arms or legs.
- Weightlifting is best if it's combined with a hardy weight-bearing exercise such as running.

Wayne Wescott, fitness research director at the South Shore YMCA in Quincy, Massachusetts, and the author of *Strength Training Past 50*, had 1,132 people, average age fifty-five, follow two weight-training programs. One group worked out twice a week and another worked out three times. They worked out at 75 percent of their maximum capacity and they used 13 different exercises for a total body workout of about 25 minutes. They also did 20 minutes of aerobic exercise.

Those who worked out three times a week gained 2.5 pounds of muscle in two months and lost 4.6 pounds of fat without dieting. That's impressive. But what's more impressive is that the group that worked out twice a week gained 2.2 pounds of muscle and lost 4.4 pounds of fat. The folks who worked out more weren't wasting their time but they weren't gaining as much ground as you'd think, either.

Is the goal to make us all look like Arnold Schwarzenegger? No. Strength training will increase the size and power in a muscle and make you proud to wear a tank top, but the benefits go beyond that. The added strength helps you stand more erect and helps stave off back problems. It helps you avoid falls. And when you do fall, the muscles make it less likely that you'll break a bone. Although women have less muscle mass then men, when both embark on a weightlifting program, the percentage of strength gain is equal. A recent study at Penn State's Center for Sports Medicine found that women increased their upper arm muscle tissue by 10 to 37 percent in six months. That's similar to what men could do during the same time.

Coming Back from a Long Layoff

You can get into great shape and then lose all the benefits of your hard work in just a matter of weeks. Studies have shown that there is a significant reduction in a person's aerobic capacity after just a two-week layoff. After as little as four weeks, you've lost half of your gains and after ten weeks you are back where you started. This happens to a lot of people when the days get shorter and the weather turns cold in the winter. They stop exercising, gain weight over the holidays, and then wonder whether they have enough ambition to start all over again. People who have stayed in shape for many years won't lose their fitness quite as fast as those who are on a boom-and-bust cycle.

One thing people don't realize is that they can cut way back on their training and still maintain their fitness. If you stop training altogether, there is an immediate and noticeable detraining effect. But if you simply back way off, you can go almost four months without losing any cardiovascular fitness. In one study, athletes who reduced the frequency and duration of their training by as much as two-thirds but maintained the intensity of the work didn't lose a step. But when athletes reduced the intensity of their training by a third or two-thirds, their cardiovascular fitness plummeted. Keep in mind that this grace period lasts only about fifteen weeks. Eventually you will start to lose some of your endurance at these greatly reduced training levels.

This is good to keep in mind if you enter a busy period in your life and you can't work out as much as you want. But beware. Don't shortchange exercise. There are a new flock of books on the market for time-starved athletes that will tell you to stay fit with jumping jacks at your desk or by getting coffee from the pot farthest from your work station, but don't succumb to the premise that you are too busy to do proper exercise. Exercise should take you away from your desk, away from the coffeepot.

Fit and Fat? Burning Extra Calories for Weight Control

You see them at open-water swims, but you'll also run into them at road races, rowing regattas, and even bike races. We're talking about top-notch athletes who are packing a little extra roll around their midsection. They are still good athletes, they're just a little chubby.

Exercise will certainly help you lose weight, but you also need to restrict the number of calories you eat. People who combine exercise with a restricted diet lose more weight and have a better chance of keep-

THE SIMPLE SIT-UP

The classic sit-up has been getting a bad rap in recent years. Some say that it can injure your back and neck and really isn't helpful anyway.

The truth is that sit-ups, which work the rectus abdominis muscles (the strips of muscle that run from the breastbone to the pelvis) and the layers of muscle that flank them, can help protect your back, enhance your physique, and improve your endurance in a wide variety of sports, from running and swimming to cross-country skiing and rock climbing. But they have to be done correctly.

The secret to a good sit-up is to isolate the abs and keep the powerful hip flexors out of the action. The best way to do this is to bend the knees 90 degrees, keep your feet flat on the floor (12–18 inches from your butt) and raise up slowly, but only part way. Stop about 6 or 12 inches off the floor, flex your abs while you hold the position, and then slowly return to the floor. You should never twist while doing the sit-up and you should quit at the slightest twinge of pain. Here are some other things to guide your sit-up work:

- Avoid specialized ab machines. Most are useless.
- Avoid high-volume, high-speed repetitions. You should start each

ing it off. The mistake a lot of people make is that they cut way back on their caloric intake and their body reacts by trying to store all those calories as fat.

FIT AND FAT?   73
BURNING
EXTRA
CALORIES
FOR WEIGHT
CONTROL

Experts at the Cooper Institute in Dallas recommend that people who want to lose weight consume 300–500 fewer calories than they expend each day. Half the deficit should come from eating less and half should come from exercising more. If you walk 4 miles in 1 hour, for instance, you'll burn 250–300 calories. If you run for a half hour at 10 minutes a mile, you'll burn the same amount. Many machines at health clubs ask you to enter your weight before you start exercising and then count your calories for you while you work out, and this can help you track your output a little better. But if you are cheating and leaning heavily on the hand rails of a stair climber, you'll actually burn up to 30 percent fewer calories than the machine says.

Exercise helps weight loss in ways that can't be calculated simply. For instance, trained muscles, even at rest, burn more energy, and that

movement slowly and visualize the abs tensing up and shortening. If a friend is nearby, have her touch those muscles while you're doing the sit-up.

- Exhale while the abs contract so you can suck the muscles inward and ensure that even the deeper muscles are getting some work. Keep the abs tense when you return to the floor.

- You can also try medicine ball drills or abdomen punching drills with some of your pugilistic pals. But wait until you've strengthened your midsection.

- Ease into it. Start out with just a few sit-ups, adding a couple a day until you can start doing sets of 15.

- Start out with your hands to your side and systematically move them closer to your head as you get stronger. After you get used to having your arms at your side, cross them at your chest. Then put them behind your head. Eventually you should be able to cross your arms behind your head and put each hand on the opposite shoulder while doing your sit-ups.

expends calories. Working muscles also have to be restocked with gly-cogen after the exercise is over, and that burns calories, too. It's also been shown that exercise improves a person's discipline, making him or her less likely to order fries with that burger. "People lose more weight than you can explain by the calories burned from exercise," says Kelly Brownell, a Yale University psychologist who studies eating disorders.

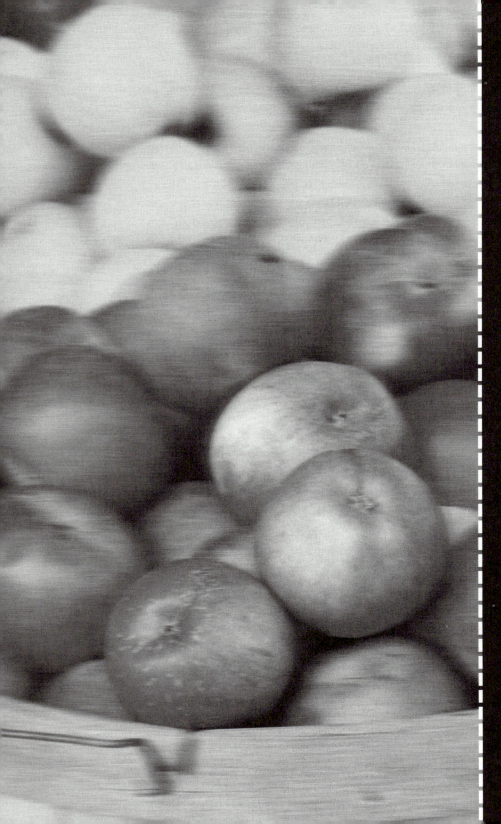

CHAPTER 5

THE CARE AND FEEDING OF AN ATHLETE

erhaps no other area of health and fitness has generated more conflicting reports, advice, and confusion than nutrition. Some doctors say vitamin supplements are good, some say they are bad. Some say cut out the salt, others say salt is good for you. A flood of new books urges people to eat a high-protein, low-carbohydrate diet, even though health professionals everywhere say most of your calories should come from complex carbohydrates, particularly if you exercise. Everybody used to say you should never eat before exercise; now you hear that if it's not an intense activity like sprinting or speed skating, it's probably a good idea to eat something to give you an extra boost of energy.

Then there is the bombardment of messages from the food makers themselves, who twist studies to serve their own needs and sell their products. Since the end of World War II, which marked the advent of our country's powerful food-processing industry, we've needed experts to tell us how to eat right and how to plan the right menu. Visitors to our country are astonished at the wide array of fresh foods found in our supermarkets—the twelve varieties of apples, the shrink-wrapped poultry, the bags of fresh and frozen vegetables—but Americans are somewhat self-conscious about this abundance. In many ways we are afraid of our food—afraid we'll eat too much of it, or not the right combinations of it, or that we'll find out the food contains mysterious bacteria or too much fat, or was prepared in a way that violated the environment or another species. We get meat that's already been seasoned or even already cooked because we're not sure what to do with the plain raw stuff. Somehow we've turned one of our chief pleasures in life—eating—into something to be leery of.

Even if you want to eat right, it seems like a daunting task that can only end in failure. There is a laundry list of vitamins and minerals the body needs to consume to stay healthy; how can you possibly eat enough of the right kind of food? When you look at the food charts and the food pyramids and the new food labels, it's enough to make you dizzy. One chart says to eat four servings of fruit and five servings of vegetables and eleven servings of cereal or bread. Then there are all those servings of beans and nuts and yogurt, and you really don't like yogurt anyway. Then this study comes out about soy or ginseng or garlic and you're trying to add all that stuff, too, and you're wondering how can I stay fit eating all this stuff.

Relax. Let's sort through some of these conflicting stories and put your diet back on the right track. It's not that hard and you may find it improves your athletic performance considerably.

Basic Nutrition

We eat so we can obtain energy and stay alive, but we also eat because the body needs certain nutrients to grow, repair itself, and replace cells that are lost through attrition and environmental mishaps. You need a varied diet that includes carbohydrates and fat for energy but also the water, protein, vitamins, and minerals to build and replace cells that die through the normal course of living.

POOR OR DECLINING PERFORMANCE CAN OFTEN BE TRACED BACK TO POOR DIET.

Vitamins and essential minerals trigger biochemical reactions that take care of a wide range of functions in our bodies, from digestion to fighting off infections to keeping our brains operating at a high level. You don't burn vitamins for energy, but you can't produce energy if they aren't in your blood. Energy production relies on the activity of enzymes, and enzymes rely on micronutrients, such as vitamins and minerals, to function properly. The brain also needs good nutrition to keep the right balance of biochemistry needed to urge the body on to athletic achievement.

Minerals such as calcium and phosphorous build, maintain, and repair bones and teeth and are essential for muscle contractions. Other minerals, including iron, are key ingredients in healthy blood that can carry a lot of oxygen to working muscles. Deficiencies of any of these will also affect your brain and nervous system. For instance a deficiency of thiamin can lead to nerve damage and the disease known as beri beri. Although beri beri is rare, a mild lack of thiamin can lead to constipation and muscle cramps—not uncommon among hard-training athletes—and should send the patient scrambling for foods rich in thiamin, including pork, ham, oranges, bran cereal, beans, watermelon, and sunflower seeds.

It's not unusual for poor or declining athletic performance to be traced back to poor diet. Slight vitamin or mineral deficiencies go unnoticed by most people, but athletes notice them because they are demanding so much more of their bodies—to produce a tremendous amount of energy and repair itself again and again. Athletes are keeping daily tabs on all their body's functions, and if one of those chemical processes is gummed up, they'll notice that something is not quite right.

Athletes tend to eat better than sedentary people, but many still aren't getting all the nutrition they need. For instance, nearly 70 percent of all runners modify their diets during training, increasing carbohydrates and protein and decreasing fat. But only a third think about vitamins. But they should be making sure they are getting the right amounts of the following:

THE IMPORTANCE OF DRINKING WATER

We can get by for several weeks without food, but we'd last only a few days without water. Our bodies are about 70 percent water—we lug 45 quarts around with us to keep the currents around our cells moving properly, control our body temperature, lubricate our organs, maintain our muscle tone, and keep our minds sharp. Even if you aren't exercising, you should be drinking eight 8-ounce glasses of water a day.

But the average American gets half that, leaving many with dry, itchy skin and a groggy feeling in the morning—classic signs of dehydration.

Athletes typically don't drink enough either, even though just a small amount of dehydration—as little as 1 percent of the body's weight—can lead to an inordinately high heart rate as the body struggles to transfer heat from contracting muscles to the skin surface. Dehydration also seems to reduce the flow of blood to the working muscles. Athletes notice the effects of this the further they get into a bout of exercise; a moderate pace will feel like a moderately difficult pace, and they'll have to slow down sooner than if they had drank enough before and during the workout. The experts advise us to drink 400–600 milliliters of water (about 17 ounces) 2 hours before exercise to give our bodies time to regulate fluid volumes in and around our cells. During exercise, you should drink as much as you sweat. Most people don't; it's common for athletes to dehydrate, losing 6 percent of their body weight. Many don't think they need water because their body isn't saying it's

- Vitamin B, B$_1$, B$_2$, and B$_6$, which all help convert carbohydrates into energy. As you increase your training, it's a good idea to increase your consumption of these vitamins by eating more whole grains, fortified cereals, meat, and beans.
- Vitamin C, which helps build collagen and increases iron absorption. A study in South Africa found that ultramarathoners who took 600 mg of vitamin C a day (10 times the recommended minimum) had a significantly lower incidence of respiratory tract infections than those on a placebo. Vitamin C is found in citrus fruits, juices, and even potatoes.
- Vitamin E, which helps reduce muscle soreness and reduces chances of heart disease (not a major problem among runners anyway). There is also evidence that vitamin E is a potent antioxidant,

thirsty, but the body's thirst mechanism is notoriously lazy. Others don't drink during exercise because they experience—or fear—gastrointestinal discomfort. But this is something you can train for: Take a lot of water with you on your runs or long cross-country ski tours and get used to drinking. Always drink more than you think you need. Some people find they will drink more if the beverage is cool and sweetened, so try that if you think it will help.

Drinking during exercise doesn't seem to be very important if you're exercising for less than an hour. A study in South Africa found that cyclists exercising for less than an hour at 85 percent effort received no benefit from drinking water; in fact, it may have hampered their performance because taking in water broke their concentration and gave them a bloated feeling.

After exercise, it's a good idea to weigh yourself to see whether you lost any weight. Every pound you dropped is equal to 2 cups of water, so drink up. Also, check the color of your urine; a dark, amber color means you're close to dehydration, and pale yellow or clear urine means you're well hydrated. Carbohydrate-enhanced drinks can not only delay fatigue brought on by low blood sugar but also accelerate the body's absorption of water. But it's important to keep the amount of carbohydrate in the drink to below 10 percent—usually between 4 percent and 8 percent. That's because higher concentrations will pull water back into the intestines and bring on dehydration even faster.

reducing the damage done by free radicals released by endurance training. You can get vitamin E from margarine, oils, seeds, and nuts, but it's best to take it in a pill form because to get 100 IU (studies showing its benefits used 400–800 IU) you'd have to eat nineteen cups of spinach or seven cups of peanuts.

- Folic acid, or folate, is being touted as the next wonder nutrient. Researchers believe it reduces the risk of colon cancer and heart disease, and might work in conjunction with vitamin B_{12} to prevent Alzheimer's disease. Although the Food and Drug Administration has ordered makers of breads, flours, pastas, and rice to fortify their products with folic acid, some experts recommend supplements. Since these are more easily stored in the body, the recommended dosage is 400 micrograms.

- Iron: Several studies have found that 40 to 80 percent of all female swimmers are anemic or iron-deficient. This may also be true among female runners. A lot of athletes don't realize they are anemic until their iron stores are depleted, and then they are looking at a recovery of several weeks. You can boost your iron consumption by eating liver, bran flakes, beans, beef, eggs, and tomato sauce. Some athletes need to take iron supplements, even though getting the extra iron from food reduces the risk of getting too much iron in your system. Vitamin C helps promote the storage of iron.

Pills Versus Meals

Because your body can't make most vitamins and minerals, it needs to get them from food. Although it might be tempting to pop a multivitamin and then head to McDonald's, experts say that's a big mistake. You need to get vitamins from food because food contains hundreds of additional nutrients, including compounds called phytochemicals, that the body needs to function at a high level. Doctors who advocate vitamin supplements tend to view them as an insurance policy for when illness, stress, or injury increases your body's need for nutrients.

Some exceptions are made for those who are older than fifty. According to the National Academy of Sciences, those fifty and older need to take synthetic supplements of vitamin B_{12}, a nutrient found in animal products, including fish, meat, and dairy food. Vitamin B_{12}, also known as cobalamin, helps maintain red blood cells and protects nerve cells. The academy also recommends that those fifty and older increase their consumption of other B vitamins, including folic acid, thiamin, and niacin, as well as vitamin D and calcium. Doctors used to tell people in this age group to reduce consumption of vitamins, but now they realize that they need vitamins as much as younger people do, if not more so. Vitamin B_{12} is needed because up to a third of all people who reach age fifty lose their ability to produce enough stomach acid to extract all the vitamin B_{12} that comes down the chute. Without enough B_{12}, people can become anemic and suffer nerve damage that leaves them demented, confused, or suffering memory problems. How much do you need? Try up to 25 micrograms per day, an amount supplied by many multivitamin pills.

GET ENOUGH FIBER.

One of the advantages of getting vitamins from food is that there is much less risk of getting too much of a particular vitamin or mineral. Your body works to maintain an optimal level of each vitamin in the blood, but sometimes gets more than it needs. Surpluses of four of the thirteen vitamins—A, D, E, and K—are stored in your body's fat, and surpluses of the nine water-soluble vitamins—vitamin C and the eight B vitamins, thiamin (B_1), riboflavin (B_2), niacin, vitamin B_6, pantothenic acid, vitamin B_{12}, biotin, and folic acid—are excreted in urine. Fat-soluble vitamins can accumulate in your body to toxic levels, so athletes who have a good diet and are also taking strong vitamin supplements run the risk of getting too much of a good thing. They're also generating some expensive pee.

For the millions of healthy Americans who take a daily multivitamin supplement, the risks of side effects are pretty small. But if you're tempted to take high-dose vitamins, thinking that more is better, think again. According to the Institute of Medicine, more than 100 milligrams of vitamin B_6 can lead to pain or numbness in limbs, more than 1,000 micrograms of folic acid can lead to nerve damage, more than 35 milligrams of niacin can cause flushing or itching, and more than 3.5 grams of choline can dangerously lower your blood pressure and make you smell like a dead fish.

Although a handful of studies have shown that you can increase endurance with large doses of C, E, and B-complex vitamins, many more studies have proven that premise false. Popping vitamins will not make up for a lack of talent or training. Your body is especially sensitive to too much vitamin A and vitamin D.

A Simple Recipe for Eating Right

With all the food pyramids, package labels, and scare reports about the fat content in everything from sandwiches to Mexican food, it's not surprising that we are a little intimidated by food these days. Not only do you have to eat the kind of food that gives you thirteen vitamins, fifteen or more minerals, and eight amino acids, but you also have to limit

CHEAT TO WIN? ARTIFICIAL SHORTCUTS TO STRENGTH AND FITNESS

Linford Christy, the 1992 100-meter gold medalist from England, swears by the stuff. So did Angel Martino, the oldest medal-winning swimmer at the 1996 Summer Games in Atlanta, who at the ripe old age of twenty-nine swam some of the fastest times of her career.

We're talking about creatine monohydrate, an ergogenic aid that is seducing huge numbers of athletes with its promise of making them stronger, faster, and more resilient.

Creatine is an amino acid produced in small amounts by the kidneys, liver, and pancreas. It's stockpiled in the muscles, where it's used to recycle ATP at a very rapid rate. The body uses the creatine phosphate system when exercise initially begins, but its primary function is to fuel rapid-fire muscle contractions during sprints and other explosive activity. Its supply is exhausted in about 10 seconds in most people.

After scientists learned that muscle cells can be juiced up with 30 percent more creatine than they normally carry, weightlifters started taking supplements and making big gains. Creatine has since been embraced by a wide variety of athletes, including swimmers and endurance athletes, who say it helps them work out harder and recover faster from their workouts. Field tests have shown that creatine buffers and regulates lactic acid, which allows you to keep going longer at a difficult pace.

Studies have shown that taking creatine every day for 5–7 days increases sprint performance by up to 5 percent and work performed in repeated sprints by up to 15 percent. Taking creatine supplements for a month or two during

your calories to 2,900 a day for men or 2,200 a day for women. What's more, you also have to figure out some percentages, like how to make sure that 58 percent of your diet is carbohydrates, 12 percent is protein, and no more than 30 percent is fat. And then there is cholesterol: Make sure you get no more than 300 mg a day. Although some of these percentages should be different for athletes—athletes have to eat more and their percentage of carbohydrates has to go up if they are in heavy training and need to replenish energy stores every day after a tough workout—their approach to eating should be pretty much the same as everybody else's.

It's no wonder, then, that many people don't get all the nutrients

training can improve sprint performance by 5 to 8 percent, and gains in strength can be as much as 15 percent. The only known side effect is increased body weight (and muscle cramping if you don't drink at least eight glasses of water a day). Older athletes should be cautious with creatine because it can overload already weakened kidneys. Creatine has been on the market only since 1993, so some unknown long-term side effects may show up in the future.

A couple of other supplements have come onto the market in recent years, including DHEA, which purportedly increases energy, improves mood, and prevents cancer and heart disease, and androstenedione, an over-the-counter supplement that converts to testosterone in the body. Elevated levels of testosterone enable athletes to work out harder and recover more quickly. Androstenedione was first developed in the 1970s by East German scientists for their Olympic athletes, and the substance has been available in this country since 1996. Manufacturers say a 100-milligram dose of androstenedione increases testosterone levels by 300 percent and lasts for about 3 hours. Although anyone can buy androstenedione, some stores refuse to stock it because of possible risks. It's also been banned by the National Football League and the International Olympic Committee, but professional baseball players use it all the time. Mark McGwire used it the year he pounded seventy home runs. Androstenedione is not as popular among endurance athletes as creatine, and that might be because it hasn't been fully tested and because many feel like it's cheating.

they need from their diets. According to the Mayo Clinic, only one person in ten regularly consumes the recommended five servings a day of fruits and vegetables, and athletes aren't innocent of that kind of transgression. Marathoner Bill Rodgers used to slather mayonnaise on leftover pizza as a preworkout meal and Frank Shorter remembers living on beer and junk food while training for the 1972 Olympics.

But eating well isn't all that hard, not in our society, where food is plentiful, varied, and cheap. Here are a few basic rules you can follow that keep you on the right track:

- Fashion a daily dining load that includes two 3-ounce cuts of lean meat, poultry, or fish; two 8-ounce glasses of milk; two cups of cooked vegetables; three large pieces of fruit; three slices of bread; one and a half cups of cereal, rice, pasta, potato, or starchy beans; and five teaspoons of butter, margarine, oil, mayonnaise, or other fat (such as salad dressing). This gives you 1,600 calories, and you can work up from there, avoiding more fat and always looking for ways to add fruits or vegetables. Nutritionist Liz Applegate, an advisor for *Runner's World* magazine, recommends that runners aim for 1,600 calories from carbohydrates every day. You can get that from five slices of bread, seven pieces of fruit, and 2 cups of cooked vegetables (4 cups uncooked).

- Always consume high–nutrient-density foods, which includes vegetables, legumes, lean meats, whole-grain breads, and fruits. These foods should be prepared with a minimal amount of fat or sugar.

- Vitamins that dissolve in water, such as B vitamins and vitamin C, escape from vegetables into cooking water or steam. Microwaving protects vitamins because it cooks vegetables quickly in little or no water. Steaming has the same effect if you use a steamer basket held above the water level. Cover the pan and cook just until tender. Largest vitamin losses stem from overcooking.

- Try to eat fish two or three times a week. Many fish, including fatty fish like salmon, include a group of fats called omega-3, which are essential in holding off heart disease and arthritis. Flaxseed oil has omega-3, too, but cooking with it kills the benefit.

- Although many nutrients are evenly distributed in food, many are not and you have to take careful steps to make sure you get them. There is no vitamin A or C in meats or breads, for instance, so you have to eat something like an orange to get your C and a carrot to get your vitamin A.
- Don't be afraid of meat. It is a valuable source of vitamins and minerals, but chances are you don't need to eat as much as you usually do. How much steak, for instance? All you need is a piece of meat the size of a deck of cards. Switch from processed meats such as bacon, ham, hot dogs, and sausages to their reduced-fat or fat-free versions. Processed meats are the second leading source of fat in Americans' diet.
- Stay away from fats and fatty foods. Just do it. Switch from 2 percent milk to 1 percent or skim. Switch from stick margarine or butter to reduced-fat tubs. Switch from ground beef to ground turkey; Americans get more saturated fat from ground beef than from all other forms of beef combined.

EATING AWAY OSTEOPOROSIS

The Institute of Medicine recommends adults ages nineteen to fifty increase calcium intake from 800 milligrams to 1,000 milligrams and that adults over age fifty-one bump it up to 1,200 milligrams. In addition to milk and dairy products, you can get calcium from black-eyed peas, steamed spinach, canned pink salmon with the bone in it, and steamed kale.

If you're buying orange juice, look for a brand that contains FruitCal, a calcium source made from calcium and two types of fruit acids. If you're going to take a pill, the National Osteoporosis Foundation recommends supplements that say "purified." Avoid calcium made from unrefined oyster shell, dolomite, or bone meal, which tends to have higher levels of lead. Calcium carbonate supplements are best taken at mealtimes, but calcium citrate preparations can be taken any time. Keep in mind that calcium content in different foods varies depending on where it comes from. For instance, skim milk in California contains 15 percent more calcium than milk from Nebraska. Food grown in different soil and mineral conditions will yield different calcium levels, too.

- When in doubt, have a second helping of pasta. Although the body's sense of hunger and satiety is extremely accurate and should be consulted regularly, some endurance athletes underestimate how much carbohydrate they need to eat. Athletes who train intensively but eat low-carbohydrate diets (only 40 percent of total caloric intake) will experience a daily decline in muscle glycogen and require 2 days or more to recover from a tough workout. When that percentage of carbohydrate is increased to 70 percent of the diet, muscle glycogen replacement is completed in 22 hours, which means they are ready to work out hard again the next day. This has been backed up by a number of studies that show that the more carbohydrates you consume, the more glycogen your muscles will store. The amount of exercise you can perform to exhaustion is directly proportional to the amount of glycogen available for exercise.

- Use alcohol in moderation. Moderate alcohol consumption increases the HDL level in the blood and helps prevent clogging of the arteries. It can also lower blood pressure. And antioxidants in red wine have been shown to reduce the risk of heart disease, although some dispute these findings and say you can get the same benefit from eating grapes. Moderate consumption is usually two 12-ounce bottles of beer or two 4-ounce glasses of wine. Keep in mind, however, that alcohol has many damaging effects: It damages the stomach lining, can cause degeneration of the liver, compromises the immune system, and interferes with the absorption of nutrients during digestion.

- Get your fiber. There are two types of fiber—soluble and insoluble—and each serves a different role. Insoluble fiber, found in wheat bran, promotes passage of material through the gut and helps protect against colon cancer. Soluble fiber, found in fruits, vegetables, and oat bran, promotes excretion of cholesterol.

- Enjoy it. Eating is one of life's principal pleasures. Many athletes stay on a training program simply because they want to feel free to drink a beer at the end of the day or eat a bowl of ice cream at night. Nothing wrong with that.

Before, During, and After Exercise: Eating to Win

BEFORE, 87
DURING,
AND AFTER
EXERCISE:
EATING
TO WIN

How much you eat before exercise depends on the time of day you are working out and how much you ate at your last meal.

If you are working out first thing in the morning, it's a good idea to nibble on something, such as a piece of fruit or some whole-wheat graham crackers. And always make sure to drink water or diluted juice to rehydrate after a night of snoring and drooling. If you're planning to exercise more than an hour, eat and drink a little bit more and bring along some sports bars or gels.

If you're working out in the evening, you can have some simple carbohydrates—a piece of fruit or something light, like half a bagel. If your workout is still 2 hours away, some protein and fat—in the form of cheese and crackers, say—are okay, too.

Many athletes worry about the type of carbohydrate they eat before exercise. What's got them concerned is a phenomenon known as rebound hypoglycemia, a condition in which certain foods stimulate insulin production, increase the rate at which muscles burn glycogen, and cause glucose levels to drop, making the athlete feel sluggish. Although some studies have discredited the idea of rebound glycemia, it's a very real phenomenon with some athletes. They head out on a long trail run, thinking they are well fed and watered, and shortly into the run they start to feel weak and shaky and start getting some flashes of light in their eyes. You don't think you can go on, but if you slow down and press ahead, your body corrects itself fairly quickly. Before long you're moving along as if nothing had happened.

It's widely accepted that if you are exercising longer than an hour it's a good idea to consume some carbohydrates mixed with water, rather than just water alone. Research also suggests it's a good idea to take on some carbs if you are doing bursts of speed over the course of a long run, ski, or ride. It's still not certain whether carbs are needed during workouts less than an hour in length.

Eating Before a Race

One of the first science-based fueling strategies to break on the exercise scene in the early 1970s was a process called carbo-loading. It required that athletes work out to exhaustion one week before a big event, like a marathon, and then go 3 or 4 days without ingesting any carbohydrates. This was grueling; these were athletes who had been training—and eating—at high levels for months and suddenly they were left feeling listless, irritable, and anxious. Of course, as they backed off their training and began loading up on pasta and rice and other carbohydrates later on in the week, their strength returned and they developed a level of confidence and strength.

Studies later showed that you didn't have to go through the depletion stage of the carbo-loading—that you could get the same level of glycogen in your blood simply by backing off from exercise and eating more carbohydrates. But many athletes stick to the old practice out of superstition or fear that they might hit 20 miles in their marathon and have no energy left.

The last meal you have before a race should be designed to ensure a normal level of blood sugar and help you avoid feeling hungry or weak before your race. You need to plan the meal so your stomach and upper bowel are empty before the race starts. Eating too much sugar an hour before the race could trigger overproduction of insulin and leave you feeling fatigued. The recommendation: Eat 2 hours before the contest and eat only foods that are easily digested. A lot of athletes prefer a nutritionally dense liquid meal to solid food.

There is also new evidence that ultraendurance athletes should boost the amount of fat in their diet, from about 30 percent to nearly 40 percent. Male cyclists who rode for 3 hours at a low intensity burned more fat for energy after being on the high-fat diet for a week than they did when 73 percent of their calories came from carbohydrates. Researchers didn't get the same results from women, but that might be because their test was only for 2 hours. The advantage of burning more fat, of course, is that you can conserve your limited supplies of glycogen and keep going longer.

Replacing Energy During Exercise

Sports bars burst on the scene many years ago but are slowly being supplanted by energy gels: packets of highly concentrated carbohydrates that quickly replace glycogen while you're on the move. One packet contains about 100 calories and approximately 25 grams of carbohydrate, and their ingredients include simple sugars (fructose or dextrose) and long-chain carbohydrates or glucose polymers. Energy gels contain no fiber, and most contain no protein. They also have fewer calories than sports bars, although many athletes prefer them because they deliver energy more quickly.

BEFORE,
DURING,
AND AFTER
EXERCISE:
EATING
TO WIN

89

Although scientific research has yet to confirm the effects of energy gels, anecdotal evidence from consumers suggests that the gels do eliminate muscle glycogen depletion and blood sugar spikes when consumed at regular intervals. For high-performance athletes such as marathon cyclists, manufacturers recommend one packet every 30 minutes taken with 8–10 ounces of water.

Gels may give endurance athletes an extra boost, but most athletes can ensure they have adequate glycogen stores by eating foods rich in carbohydrates before and after exercise. Energy gels are best for endurance athletes who are exercising for more than 1.5 hours.

EAT FOODS RICH IN CARBOHYDRATES BEFORE AND AFTER EXERCISE.

The Glycogen Window: Restocking Your Energy Stores

How quickly after exercise should you start eating again? If it was a short workout, you probably didn't use up much of the glycogen stored in your body and you don't have to worry about replenishing it. If it was a long, exhaustive workout, however, you need to eat within a 2-hour period known as the glycogen window. During that period, the body will replace glycogen 50 percent faster than if you wait more than 2 hours. If you don't eat, you'll feel sluggish the next day and won't perform well if you try to work out again. Many athletes try to eat within 15–30 minutes of their workout; others don't feel like eating right away and wait awhile.

Some studies suggest that protein and carbohydrates together replace glycogen stores more quickly. Here's where energy gels won't do you much good. Eating a bagel or cereal with milk would do the trick better.

Athletes who have been working hard say they feel suffused with contentment while eating their postworkout snacks. They can practically feel the blood delivering energy to their muscles. Don't be surprised, though, if you break into a sweat an hour or so after eating; that's a sign your body is replenishing your glycogen stores, a process that burns up some calories.

DON'T BE FOOLED BY THE PROMISE
OF MEDICINAL HERBS

Since 1994, when Congress changed the Food and Drug Administration's regulation of nutritional supplements, the health supplement industry has grown to a $6-billion-a-year business. Up to a third of all Americans take daily vitamin supplements and almost three-quarters take vitamins occasionally. In addition, Americans are spending more than $700 million a year on herbal remedies, even though there is little evidence that these supplements do any good. In fact, there is good reason to avoid herbal concoctions. Some of the products have dangerous side effects, others aren't as potent as their labels claim, and there is no government regulation or solid scientific research being done on any of these products.

A study of a dozen poison control centers around the country found that nearly 25 percent of the people who called the centers after using herbal products had gotten sick as a result of ingesting the supplements. Two people died of heart attacks, including a fifteen-year-old soccer player who had taken a product containing ephedra. A ginseng user suffered brain hemorrhaging. There were also several cases of people having seizures or falling into comas, and people who suffered heart abnormalities, liver dam-

age, fevers, and allergic reactions.

What's fueling this growth of herbal supplements is an advertising machinery that touts products as "the most powerful nutritional force in the universe" and other wild claims that manufacturers never have to prove. Critics of herbal supplements note that there is little incentive on the part of manufacturers to commission expensive clinical trials on their products if they don't have to.

An estimated one in three Americans with chronic disease looks to herbal medicines for help. But buyers may be getting more than they bargained for. In 1998, researchers analyzed herbal supplements called Chinese black balls after five people developed stomach pain or drowsiness. The small black pills are sold under names such as Miracle Herb and Tung Shueh, for conditions including arthritis and liver and kidney problems. Although the only ingredients listed in Chinese black balls are herbs, the analysis revealed the presence of non-steroidal anti-inflammatory drugs and antianxiety medications such as Valium and Librium.

Still, herbs are the basis for many of our most helpful medicines, including aspirin, morphine, and digitalis. And scientists are still making discoveries; the new

BEFORE, 91
DURING,
AND AFTER
EXERCISE:
EATING
TO WIN

anticancer drug paclitaxel is derived from the bark and needles of the Pacific yew tree. But doctors suggest that you use these precautions: Don't use herbal remedies for serious illnesses, don't give herbs or other dietary supplements to children, and don't use herbal supplements if you're pregnant or trying to get pregnant. To avoid interactions with other medications, tell your doctor about all supplements you take.

Here are some of the top supplements and some of their purported advantages and disadvantages:

• **Saint John's wort:** With antidepressants being three of the top ten drugs in the United States, it's not surprising many people have turned to more natural remedies for the blues. And increasingly the plant of choice is Saint John's wort, a yellow-flowered plant with the Latin name *Hypericum perforatum.* The ancient Greeks thought it could ward off evil spirits, but in Europe, where it has been popular for fifteen years, folks know it as just a good antidepressant; German doctors prescribe it 3 million times a year—25 times as often as Prozac. Although more clinical study is needed on its effectiveness, initial studies have been very promising. One study of 3,250 patients with mild to moderate depression found that 80 percent either felt better or were free of depression after just four weeks. The optimum dosage is 300 milligrams of the herb three times a day. But beware: a survey by the *Los Angeles Times* found that six of the top ten brands of Saint John's wort had less potency than indicated on the label. Ask your health food store proprietor for assurances that the brand you're buying is legitimate. There might be some side effects; 2.4 percent of the 3,250 patients reported restlessness, gastrointestinal irritation, and mild allergic reactions. Some sheep put on the supplement have gotten sick or died from exposure to the sun, but there have been no human reports of phototoxicity.

• **Garlic:** Thirty clinical studies have shown that one to two cloves a day (or its pill equivalent) can reduce cholesterol in the blood by 15 percent—enough to reduce the risk of heart attack by 30 percent. It

(Continued on next page)

can also help prevent blood clots, and hundreds of studies have suggested that it can prevent (but not cure) many forms of cancer.

- **Ginkgo:** It's widely used in Europe to treat strokes and poor circulation to the brain, but it increases blood flow to the penis as well as to the brain. In one study, fifty men with erection impairment got 240 milligrams of gingko daily for nine months and 78 percent regained their erections. Side effects can include gastrointestinal problems, headaches, and allergic skin reactions.
- **Ginseng:** There are a lot of claims about ginseng, but the only likely effect is that it increases sexual desire. Several Asian and Russian studies back that up, but American scientists remain skeptical. Dr. Andrew Weil, M.D., who worked for fifteen years as a research associate in ethnopharmacology at the Harvard Botanical Museum, recommends ginseng as a tool for enhancing immunity. But he warns that some products that claim to provide the healing powers of ginseng actually contain little or no ginseng. You can be assured

of finding the real thing by buying the whole ginseng root, but that can be expensive. Weil advises consumers to look for ginseng products that are clearly labeled and contain concentrations of ginsenosides, the active chemical compound in ginseng.

- **Echinacea:** This herb is really popular during the cold and flu season and is purported to boost your immune system and ward off diseases. Studies show that a regimen of vitamin C, echinacea, and zinc lozenges can help keep a cold from developing into something worse and shorten its lifespan. Continued use decreases the effect, and some people have had allergic reactions to it.
- **Black and green tea:** There is strong scientific evidence that these beverages—made from tea leaves, not herbs—protect against many forms of cancer. They have more antioxidant power than fruits and vegetables, and may reduce the risk of heart disease. The antioxidants in tea, called plant polyphenols, are similar to those found in spinach, broccoli, tomatoes, and other fruits and vegetables.

CHAPTER 6

HOW EXERCISE IMPROVES YOUR MOOD AND YOUR BRAIN

There is something that people fear more than losing their physical strength, something they fear even more than dying: losing their minds. And mental deterioration as we age seems as inevitable to many of us as our physical deterioration. Just as we expect our MHR to drop, our race times to slow down, and our aches and pains to become more nagging, we also expect to become a little more forgetful, maybe a little less nimble in our thinking.

But a new wave of studies is forcing many of us to reconsider our long-held beliefs about how age affects our brains. And not surprisingly, an increasing number of researchers are stepping forward to say that exercise—both mental and physical—is a person's best insurance for heading off the steady fraying of the mind that many associate with aging. The best stimulant for your brain—the best way to regenerate nerve cells lost to age and stressful living—is to get your blood pumping. Rats that train on a treadmill develop more capillaries—and more blood flow—to their brains. Studies on humans have shown that people who exercise generate more new brain cells than those who don't.

Neurologists are now looking at the aging brain with the same new attitude that physiologists are looking at aging bodies—with the belief that there doesn't have to be the kind of deterioration we always thought was inevitable. Just as physical aging studies are turning from sedentary people to fit people, neurologists are paying more attention to older people who have never lost cognitive function. And what they are finding is just as heartening: "Older people can continue to have extremely rich and healthy mental lives," says Dr. Antonio Damasio, head of the Department of Neurology at the University of Iowa.

In fact, recent studies have consistently shown that—contrary to previously held beliefs—the IQ of elderly people does not decrease with age. Scientists now have a way of scanning the activity of the brain, and they've watched in wonderment at the flexibility of the aging mind. Challenged, put to the test, an old brain responds just like a new brain: It grows new connections between brain cells. A Harvard study of 1,003 physicians between the ages of twenty-eight and ninety-two found that mental agility is retained more often by men who continue to work after age sixty-five. In a separate study, researchers at UCLA tested thirty-five intellectually gifted men at intervals between ages seventy and eighty and found that 77 percent increased the size of their working vocabularies during that decade. These findings back up the work done by William Greenough at the University of Illinois, who found that animals that are challenged intellectually can grow new synaptic connections at any age. The brain, just like the rest of the body, needs exercise.

It's true that many aging minds get frayed at the edges, but disease is a greater cause than anyone previously thought possible. However, exercise could help in that regard as well. A 1998 study at Case Western Reserve University in Cleveland suggested that life-long, regular physical exercise might prevent Alzheimer's disease. Alzheimer's is the most common cause of dementia in the United States and afflicts an estimated 4 million people. But neurologists who studied 126 people (average age seventy-seven) with Alzheimer's and a comparable group of healthy people found that the healthy people reported significantly more physical activity during the forty years between their twentieth and fifty-ninth birthdays. The finding agreed with earlier studies that found staying physically, mentally, and socially active helps protect against Alzheimer's.

THE BEST STIMULANT FOR YOUR BRAIN IS TO GET YOUR BLOOD PUMPING.

The other great destroyer of brain cells is stress. When monkeys who are accustomed to living quietly by themselves are tossed into a small cage with other monkeys, their brains' cell production rate falls off within an hour. So reduce your stress and you'll keep your brain's cell production factory clicking along, right? That's easier said than done. Exercise takes care of some of the stress for you, but what about the rest?

Experts in psychiatry and neurology suggest that we pull ourselves up by our own bootstraps and cultivate a sense that we are charting our own course through life. Shrinks call it self-efficacy. You control your fate, not someone else. The secret is to reframe stress and treat it as though it's a challenge, not a burden.

"It's not whether you experience stress," says Marilyn Albert, a professor of psychiatry and neurology at Harvard University, "it's your attitude toward it."

How Exercise Stimulates Your Mind

Perhaps nothing is more effective at reorganizing your brain and re-ducing the stress of modern life than exercise—vigorous, disciplined training. Study after study has shown that exercise elevates your mood, sparks your creativity, and improves your problem-solving skills—all the things you need to control a hectic life and put your time to better use. Yet the primary reason people don't exercise is because they say they don't have time for it. It's a paradox. You don't have time for the one thing you need to do to make better use of your time.

Kim Layton, a fifty-six-year-old engineer who took up running at age fifty and broke 3 hours in the marathon six years later, sometimes encounters his coworkers in the parking lot at lunchtime. Layton is

HOW TO IMPROVE YOUR MEMORY

Doctors have a couple of ways of telling whether memory loss is serious. If the patient comes to them worried about his or her memory, it's usually not something serious. If a spouse or a relative goes to the doctor with those concerns, it could be something to worry about. If you say, "Ah ha. That's right!" when you're reminded of the name you forgot, you're probably okay.

Researchers have noticed that people's concern about how much they recall seems directly related to the explosion of information available to us; we're trying to cram too much knowledge into our brains and consequently some very basic stuff—like where we parked the car—is getting nudged out. One study at Utah State University suggests that exercise can help boost your memory. In that study, people who took a nine-week water aerobics course scored better on a memory test than a similar non-exercising group. There's also evidence that a good night's sleep will help your recollection; those whose dreams are interrupted don't seem to process memories from the day before as well. And according to the Human Nutrition Research Center in North Dakota, there is some evidence that the minerals zinc and boron can help revitalize your memories. Zinc is included in many daily vitamins, and you can also get it in meat and oysters. The study on boron found that men who consumed 3.5 milligrams of boron a day—the amount you can get in three apples or a similar supply of prunes, dates, raisins, or peanuts—scored much higher on memory tests.

heading out to the nearby bike path for a 10-mile run while his coworkers are heading off to a restaurant. "They'd say, 'Wow, it's great you have time to do that, to exercise.' And I'd say, 'I have the same time you have. I've just decided to use it differently.'"

Countless studies have shown a link between exercise and good moods. Scientists at Duke University Medical Center put fifty-five people on a vigorous treadmill workout for 15 minutes and 82 percent of them scored lower in feelings of depression, anger, tension, fatigue, and confusion. A different survey by the National Health and Nutrition Examination Survey found that sedentary people were three times more likely to be depressed than their exercising counterparts.

Most people feel calm and have a sense of well-being after they

If you're worried about your memory slipping somewhat, try these exercises recommended by the National Institute of Neurological Disorders and Stroke:

- **Pay attention.** Your mind isn't a video recorder. If you weren't concentrating on something—what your wife said about that red light coming on in the car or where you last put your car keys—chances are you won't remember it.
- **Rehearse and repeat.** You're in the car driving home from work and you get a great idea for the book you are writing. You can't write it down now, but it's still important. So repeat the idea to yourself a couple of times before you get home. It will be there when you get to a pad.
- **Chunk.** Group a ten-digit phone number into three chunks.
- **Visualize.** Go back to the idea-filled drive home, only this time it's a phone call you need to make. In addition to rehearsing, you can also visualize a telephone installed on your front door. When you see the door, you'll remember the phone and the call you want to make.
- **Word games.** You've used these all through your life. How did you remember the names of the Great Lakes? HOMES (Huron, Ontario, Michigan, Erie, and Superior). Rhymes and word associations (spring forward, fall back) also help.
- **Get organized.** Most people get disorganized because they feel like

(Continued on next page)

exercise. Their anxieties are tempered or gone completely, and they are more invigorated, more productive at work, and more interested in sex. One theory is that the exercising body releases beta-endorphin, a natural substance that is hundreds of times more potent than morphine, within 12 minutes of the start of exercise. Another theory is that exercise triggers the release of serotonin, a brain chemical that brings on a powerful sense of well-being and increased appetite. Serotonin is an important neurotransmitter involved in emotions and thinking, and low levels of it in the brain have been linked to depression, anxiety, suicide, aggression, and bulimia.

Exercise also enhances creativity. Researchers writing in the *British Journal of Sports Medicine* studied the responses of sixty-three people

they don't have the luxury of the time it takes to organize a drawer or filing cabinet. Find the time. It saves you time in the long run.

- **Use external aids.** Keep an appointment book. But just one. Keeping two will only mean each one is incomplete. Also, maintain a "take-away spot"—a portion of the kitchen counter where you always put your car keys, purse, or wallet upon entering the house.

- **Keep doing crossword puzzles.** By the time you reach your fifties, you have three times the vocabulary you had in your twenties, and you'll be better at crossword puzzles. Relish that and keep doing the puzzles; research shows they help

your brain develop nerve junctions, which pass along information and keep your brain sharp.

- **Marry someone smarter than you.** Studies show spouses who do this maintain or improve their brainpower as they age.

- **Use emotional tags.** Women find this particularly useful because they are better at detecting emotion. If you want to remember the name of a restaurant, remember how you felt the last time you ate there. To help remember a person's name, recall the emotion you read in that person's face—the reassuring smile he gave you or the perturbed expression that led you to believe he was tormented by something.

who took part in aerobic workouts (high-impact exercise) or aerobic dance (low-impact exercise) for 25 minutes. Participants were asked to come up with unusual uses for everyday objects—in this case tin cans and cardboard boxes. Responses were scored on number, flexibility, and originality, and researchers found that the participants' creative thinking was sparked by exercise and wasn't necessarily linked to their moods, previously thought to be a primary force behind creativity. Dance proved a better stimulus than the workout, possibly because it is less regimented and more likely to release a stream of consciousness.

EXERCISE ENHANCES CREATIVITY.

There is also a great deal of evidence that exercise affects your mental health. One study in Alameda County, California, found that people with high activity levels had less risk of depression than those who were less active. And in a study of Harvard alumni, depression rates were lower among those who were more physically active. Alumni involved in sports had only half the risk of suicide.

Those who are under a lot of stress must clear their minds of their problems during exercise or the workout won't do as much good. In a University of Georgia study, fourteen highly stressed women were placed in four different situations: One group studied while cycling on a stationary bike, another rode the bikes without textbooks, a third just studied, and a fourth sat on the bikes and did nothing. The only cyclists who became less anxious were those who rode without studying, leading researchers to conclude the exercise is most effective if you try to leave your troubles behind. If you're still obsessing about your boss during your run, you will still feel stress after it's over.

Mind Games: Using Mental Powers to Improve Fitness

Training can help your mind, but you can also use your mind to improve your performance in a race or your next workout. You can do this by developing some mental tricks that allow you to improve your attitude, focus your energy, and train your mind to control your body better. It's called performance psychology, and although it's often used by Olympic-caliber athletes, recreational athletes will find it beneficial, too.

Consider the case of Roger Bannister. Back in the early 1950s, Bannister and Gunder Haegg were the best milers in the world. Of the two, Haegg was the more consistent winner, and many track aficionados believed Haegg had more talent and raw ability.

But it is Roger Bannister we all remember because Bannister was the first man to break 4 minutes in the mile. The reason wasn't because Bannister was physically stronger than Haegg, but that he was mentally tougher.

Haegg had read somewhere that breaking 4 minutes was beyond a human's physical ability, and he came to believe that. Bannister, on the other hand, believed the barrier could be broken and he set out to do it. He trained hard for it and again and again pictured himself breaking the tape in a time that started with the number 3. Haegg himself conceded the race a month before Bannister broke the record. "I think Bannister is the man to beat 4 minutes," Haegg wrote. "He uses his brains as much as his legs."

On May 6, 1954, Bannister ran 3:59.4 on the Iffley Road track in Oxford, a feat many consider to be the greatest athletic achievement in the century. It is a story of persistence and skill, but it is also a lesson in the power of self-confidence. Nearly fifty years later, Bannister's run continues to serve as a metaphor for the glory that comes from challenging yourself and visualizing your success. "To get the most out of yourself, not just in running but in all your life's activities, set difficult goals that you believe you can achieve," William Morgan of the American College of Sports Medicine once said. "Without that belief all the training in the world won't work."

Researchers who have interviewed successful athletes have found that most have similar traits. They set many goals for themselves, and they have a knack for setting difficult goals that are also achievable. They set short-term goals and long-term goals and they work diligently toward them. What this does is keep them focused on what they are trying to achieve, but it also sets them up for success: By having many goals, they feel assured of meeting at least some of them, and this builds self-confidence.

They also have vision. Visualizing is the process of reviewing what is before you, whether it is a race or a workout, and picturing yourself doing it smoothly and effortlessly. Make the vision as detailed as possible, breaking the event or race down into parts that have smells, tastes, and colors. Even after you've started the effort, return to your vision from time to time, picturing what the next stage of the race will be.

Successful athletes—athletes who meet their goals, not necessarily those who win the race—also have the ability to see obstacles as challenges and not something that will defeat them. They are optimists, and they can dismiss negative thoughts fairly quickly. Many runners find they have trouble sleeping the night before a big race, and many allow that to affect their performance the next day. Others won't let a few fitful hours pollute their heads. They are people like Tor Aanenson, a fifty-eight-year-old Norwegian runner who ran an astonishing 2:34.20 marathon in the fifty-five to fifty-nine age group. "I have learned this much," Aanenson says, "races are won or lost in the weeks and months of training before. I don't worry about pre-race routines."

It's also important to keep your perspective. If you have failed to achieve a goal, analyze what happened and look for ways to overcome

MORE WAYS TO IMPROVE BRAIN FUNCTION

Nutritional supplements and elixirs promising to stimulate your mind have flooded the health-food market in recent years, and dozens of studies are under way for drugs that some day could improve your ability to learn and remember. But most of these claims or drugs are largely untested, and until they are, it's best to keep things simple. Research has shown that some of the things you can do to improve your brain function, in addition to exercise and intellectual stimulation, include the following:

- **Drinking a lot of water.** Eight 8-ounce glasses a day will help purify the blood going to your brain, which has more fluid than any other organ.
- **Getting foot massages.** They triple the flow of blood to the brain.
- **Using the scent of peppermint.** Peppermint increases positive brain waves for learning.
- **Testing different ideas.** Innovative thinking builds the brain faster than pat, predictable answers that have worked in the past. Even incorrect ideas will assist you here.

the problem. Focus on the issue, not the emotion or the perception that you failed. Another way to keep your perspective is to remember that this is supposed to be fun and that there is more to life than breaking 37 minutes for a 10-kilometer run.

Heinz Liesen, the national team doctor for the German soccer team that went to the World Cup in 1986 and 1990, understood that concept as well as anyone. Although his athletes were used to training fifty weeks a year for 3 to 4 hours a day, a key ingredient in Liesen's regimen involved low-intensity recuperative training that included days of total rest. Liesen also worked with his athletes to increase their creativity. He got them away from television and taught them handcrafts or foreign languages and took them to museums. The results were very impressive and lent credence to Liesen's belief that exercise levels and creative mental activity worked together to modulate health and per-

HOW TO SLOW DOWN THE PACE OF YOUR LIFE

Many doctors believe there are three things you need to do to prolong your life and make it more productive and healthy: exercise, eat right, and relax.

"Relaxation can definitely help you age better. It's important for preventing a wide variety of disorders and for increasing your effectiveness and efficiency in life," says Frank J. McGuigan, director of the Institute for Stress Management at the United States International University in San Diego.

Sounds simple, but a lot of people in this day and age have forgotten how to relax. They can try—but after a 10-hour work day that includes meetings, schedules, working on fast-paced computers,

scrambling to put together a dinner, and then carving out some quality time with the kids, all many people have energy for is crashing on the couch to watch TV. Weekends are often as carefully scheduled as the weekdays.

If you don't give yourself time to relax and unwind, you'll eventually start feeling crabby, tired, and worn out. Your frenetic lifestyle will catch up to you in the form of ulcers, migraines, high blood pressure, cardiovascular disease, and other problems. According to one study, eight in ten people who see a primary care physician are suffering from some kind of stress-related symptom.

Some people equate exercise with

formance. That's why it's important to not throw yourself completely into your training. Keep your hobby. Keep your perspective.

The Epidemic of Stress

The Buddhists call them hungry ghosts. They are spirits who were stingy and greedy in life and now wander the world yearning for the peace possessions can't provide and money can't buy.

In many ways we are a nation of hungry ghosts. Our divorce rate is 50 percent and the number-one prescription drug is Prilosec, an ulcer drug. Three of the top ten prescription drugs are prescribed for depression. A 1995 Gallup Poll that surveyed people from eighteen nations found that "a blanket of pessimism about the future seems to cover the world." There are as many as 20 million clinically depressed people in the United States, and many more suffer from dysthymia, a

leisure, but it's not. Proper training may help you relax, but it shouldn't take the place of just letting your mind wander. You need to play, to tinker. Sometimes the best time to do this is just after you've worked out, when you've already released tension and your mind is open and receptive to new ideas.

"Our minds are wired to look for new stuff," says Jane M. Healy, author of *Endangered Minds: Why Our Children Don't Think and What We Can Do About It.* "Without it, life starts to disappear in a rut. Variety keeps us awake, attentive, coaxes our minds to work and keeps our brains growing through a lifetime."

Read the local entertainment calendars and take the time to visit that museum you've driven by a thousand times, or take your kids to a Renaissance Fair. Take up a new sport, preferably one that takes you away from the hubbub of your daily life. Sometimes the pleasure comes from caring for animals or helping the environment or the less fortunate.

"The hardiest, most vital people tend to be pleasure-loving, pleasure-seeking, pleasure-creating people," says Dr. David Sobel, coauthor of *Healthy Pleasures.* "They enjoy many small daily pleasures, from the sensual to the intellectual to helping others. They expect each day to feel good."

mild form of depression that leaves people functioning in a chronically grumpy state of mind.

Part of the problem is that technology has bred a generation of "time stackers": people who see time as a commodity and try to get the most out of that investment. They balance the checkbook while they are cooking dinner and watching TV. They hold conference calls on their car phones while commuting to work, listening to the news, and eating breakfast. For many, being busy and seeming rushed is a status symbol, a measure of their importance. But that kind of stress leads to anxiety and anger, which raises levels of adrenaline, stress hormones, and blood pressure, affecting the heart and the immune system. And it leaves you with a sense that you will never get everything done, which itself gives way to an overall sense of numbness. "Everyone is talking about this problem," says stress management expert Richard Carlson, coauthor of *Slowing Down to the Speed of Life.* "It's to the point where I don't know what's going to happen if we don't slow down our way of thinking. We'll explode."

Job-related stress and all the illness that comes with it costs U.S. companies an estimated $200 billion a year, according to the American Institute of Stress and the American Psychological Association. More and more workers are filing worker's compensation claims against employers they say have heaped a debilitating amount of stress on them.

The quick pace and heavily scheduled nature of our lives today has triggered what some say is an epidemic of memory loss in middle-aged Baby Boomers. People in their forties and fifties are nervously calling their memory lapses "senior moments"—and by some anecdotal measurements, they are on the rise. "Successful, intelligent, middle-aged Baby Boomers seem to be losing their minds in great numbers," a *USA Today* article noted ominously in the summer of 1998. "Homes are full of people who can't remember what day to put out the trash."

Another reason might be that men and women both go through hormonal changes at midlife that are signaled by irritability, hot flashes, and short-term memory lapses. Some of this can be treated with hormonal treatments—women get estrogen and the men get testosterone—but the best way to deal with it is with exercise. "Try to lead a healthy life," says

neurologist David Pilgrim of Harvard Pilgrim Health Care in Boston.
"Get good exercise, good nutrition, no excess of alcohol and try to find
time to do what is important to you."

And how do you accomplish all that? A lot of people are offering up advice on the subject. Several books have made their way onto the best-seller list—from *Don't Sweat the Small Stuff* to *Simple Abundance* to *The Joy of Not Working.* The consensus seems to be that people need to strip down their lives somewhat—they need to quit charging through life like the traffic light just turned yellow. They need to start tasting their food again.

VIGOROUS, DISCIPLINED TRAINING REDUCES STRESS AND ELEVATES YOUR MOOD.

Geoffrey Godbey, a professor of leisure studies at Penn State, says you need to own less, do less, and say "no" more often. He, like many others who have studied the phenomenon, believes people spend too much time worrying about tomorrow or what happened yesterday, and that greater happiness exists in the present—in the moment you are in right now, the moment, according to the Buddhists, "where life takes place." Godbey likes to sit on his porch and watch the twilight deepen. "Sometimes you have to let things happen, rather than make them happen."

Others offer similar advice, suggesting that our national obsession with work, money, and productivity leads to physical and mental problems and vacuous lives. The irony, they say, is that it is the employee who works regular hours, has interests outside of work, and takes pleasure in the simple things in life who ends up being more productive than his workaholic counterpart. Their advice: Take up a hobby that doesn't require big bucks, like exercise. Take up walking or running. Try sewing or needlepoint. Get focused and get unfocused. Lose yourself once in a while. Ernie Zelinksi, author of *The Joy of Not Working,* calls people with balanced lives "peak performers"—people whose jobs serve them rather than the other way around.

No one knows the art of living in the moment better than children. That's all they know (until they learn differently). So when you take your kids to the zoo and they want to hang around the giraffe pen a while, hang with them and don't hurry them along. Let your kids set the pace once in a while. If you're on a hike and they want to stop and examine a worm on the trail, kneel down in the dirt with them. You might learn something.

Richard Carlson, the author of *Celebrate Your Child* and another advocate for living in the moment, recommends you stop for a minute every hour, no matter where you are, and absorb everything around you—the vibration of the car, the complex cacophony of your office, the sound the wind makes through the trees outside your bedroom window. Listen to the thumping of your own heart. Chances are it won't be beating as hard at the end of that minute.

That's a Good One: The Role of Humor

Don't underestimate the value of laughter and good humor in promoting emotional well-being and good aging. A good sense of humor has been shown in studies to help improve our social relationships and actually promotes better health by countering the effect of stress hormones and bolstering the immune system. Laughter has also been shown to have a positive effect on our cardiovascular and skeletal-muscular systems. You read that right. One study in 1988 concluded that 20 seconds of a good belly laugh is the equivalent of 3 minutes of hard rowing. You laugh, but it's true.

Studies show that people who catastrophize—who see misfortune as part of a global scheme that eventually nails everyone—are more likely to die before they are sixty-five, particularly men. These people are pessimists—victims, people who don't take responsibility for their own decisions—and they tend to be paralyzed by their own problems, socially estranged, and prone to making poor decisions. "Being in the wrong place at the wrong time might be the result of a pessimistic lifestyle," researchers said. The experience of these people doesn't necessarily recommend a life of blind optimism. But the truth is that if you get a lemon you usually can find a recipe for lemonade nearby. If you treat life as a learning experience, even your misfortunes can be used to your advantage.

Still, it's not realistic to believe anyone can be perfectly content. You can embrace simple abundance, join a Buddhist monastery, and start training for a 3-hour marathon, but you're still going to have your moments. If we didn't want more, what would drive us to become better people, to pursue art or religion? It's true that there are more negative emotions than positive ones—"there are more dangers than opportunities," explains psychiatrist Randolph Nesse of the University of Michigan—but most people give themselves a 7 on a scale of 10 in contentment. We adapt and we become happy at some level, the experts say. It's part of survival. The backdrop you pick for your portrait should be one of contentment and happiness, but remember that it is still just a backdrop. It is the surface from which our sadness, anger, and disappointment emerge and stand out for us, letting us know they are aberrant and need to be dealt with. That's life. That's how we know something is wrong, that we still have something to learn.

FINDING WORKOUT PARTNERS

Although most beginning exercisers prefer to work out alone, many eventually find that exercising with another person or in groups is a great way to maintain their motivation and to learn more about style and technique. Many older athletes find, sometimes to their surprise, that their peers aren't competitive and just like to have some company during their workouts.

An increasing number of organizations can help you find other people to work out with. For instance, many towns have active Arthritis Foundation and Leukemia Foundation offices that put together training groups each year. These are usually twenty-week group training programs. Participants pay $100, raise a few thousand more from sponsors, and then begin training for a specific race, such as the Honolulu Marathon. All their expenses to the race are paid, but what's really nice is that many of these training programs feature both walking and running, and you don't have to be an elite athlete to sign up. No one likes to disappoint a sponsor, so the success rate is very high.

Some other ideas for finding workout partners:

- The Road Runners Club of America, based in Alexandria, Virginia, promotes running and walking and has about 600 clubs and 160,000 members nationwide. Contact them to find out whether there is a club close to you.

(Continued on next page)

- Most running shoe stores have weekly training runs or walks that welcome athletes from all ability levels. This is a great way to meet potential training partners who have similar exercise schedules, but it's also a great way to learn new training routes or to push yourself harder than you normally do. Many regions also have active Sierra Clubs that sponsor free hikes, mountain bike rides, and cross-country ski trips.

- The American Running and Fitness Association (ARFA) has a program called Exercise Across America in which people pick a state to exercise across and then begin accumulating the miles they need to cross that state successfully. Simple formulas help you translate different activities, from golf to aerobic dance, into miles, and the ARFA will help you set up an individual program or a group exercise program at your place of work. Prizes are awarded to people who cross their chosen states. This program helps you stay motivated by helping you set reasonable goals (if you're just starting out, you can pick Rhode Island's 27 miles for your first goal), forcing you to keep records (you get a daily log sheet to track your miles), and giving you the recognition you need.

- The Fifty-Plus Fitness Association is a nonprofit international organization that helps older adults exercise more. The group holds fitness and social events and an annual Fitness Weekend, complete with workshops and races. The group headquarters is in Palo Alto, California, at (650) 323-6160. You can check out their Web site at fitness@ix.netcom.com.

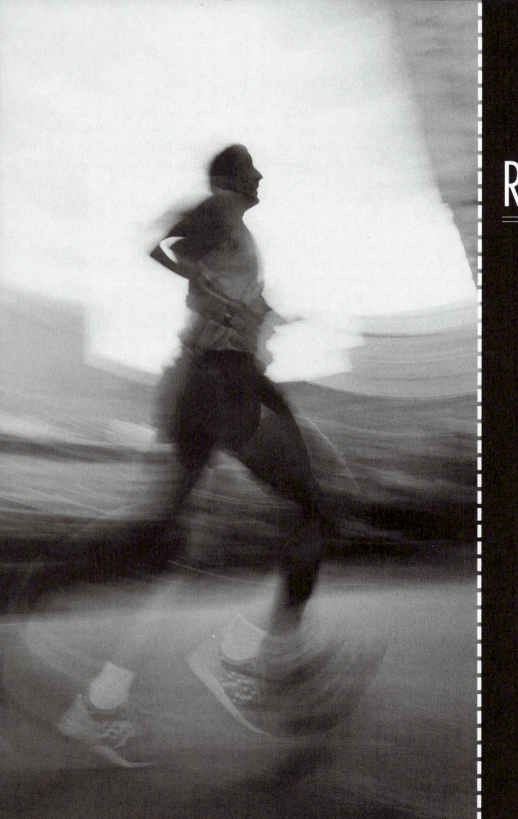

CHAPTER 7

RUNNING

For a while it seemed like everybody was running. Dr. Kenneth Cooper got people started in the late 1960s with his books on aerobics and then American Frank Shorter won the Olympic marathon in Munich in 1972 and got even more people inspired. By the mid-1980s, when the first wave of Baby Boomers started turning forty, running's popularity seemed to peak.

But now the folks who track our habits say that the running boom has fizzled. Those Baby Boomers are now looking at fifty, and running is losing its allure. "They've given up on it," Geoffrey Meredith, president of a big demographics firm in California, proclaimed in late 1998. "They are having wear and tear on their bodies."

Indeed, the knock against running in recent years is that it gives the body too much of a pounding. All those miles and all that trauma to knees, hips, and ankles. Runners have tried orthotics, knee braces, and antipronation shoes, but nothing seems to work. According to one estimate, 30 million people in the United States run and about 70 percent of them will incur an injury at some point that will prevent them from running for at least a week. That seems pretty staggering. Why would you take up a sport in which the odds of injury are so high?

Because sometimes statistics can be misleading.

The truth is that people who run regularly throughout their lives don't suffer any more bone and joint problems than those who do nothing. In one of the longest studies of runners ever conducted, researchers at Stanford University found that even runners in their sixties and seventies who had run for years and logged thousands of miles showed no undue signs of wear and tear on their joints. In fact, the runners in the study reported 20 percent less muscle and joint pain than those who didn't run at all.

The eight-year study followed the health of 451 members of a runners' club and 330 nonrunners, all between the ages of fifty and seventy-two. Not only did the runners show less joint pain and swelling, but their death rate was lower, they were leaner, and they took fewer medications than the nonrunning group. The runners' bone density was higher and they had a third as many disabilities. It turns out all those injuries attributed to running would be more accurately attributed to training mistakes, like running hard before you're warmed up properly, stretching too hard, or wearing ill-fitting shoes. That's not running, that's the runner.

Even the claim that running is losing its popularity can be disputed. The Road Running Information Center in Santa Barbara, California, claims that participation in the nation's top 100 road races is increasing a steady 3 to 5 percent a year. In 1980, those races had 350,000 finishers. By 1996, there were more than 1 million. According to the Sporting Goods Manufacturers Association, the number of frequent running participants (those running more than 3 days a week) has grown to 32.4 million, although others put the total at more than 50 million.

One thing you can say with some certainty is that runners are getting older. There are no running heroes—no Jim Ryuns or Steve Prefontaines—on the scene to inspire younger athletes to take up running. Consequently, much of the growth is coming from thirty-five- to forty-year-olds—"that age when you suddenly realize you don't get a free ride to health and you're going to have to work to stay healthy," says Clark Ensz, a veteran runner and race director in Kansas.

LOOK FOR OPPORTUNITIES TO RUN ON GRASS, OR EVEN DIRT, RATHER THAN PAVEMENT.

Why You Should Run

Running is the simplest exercise, something you can do anywhere and anytime. You can run on city streets, on the frozen turf of a local golf course, or on a breathtaking single-track trail up a mountain in a wilderness area. With the advent of high-tech, lightweight snowshoes, you can even run on the snow. Safety treads that slip over your running shoes make running on ice a little safer than it once was. If you don't want to deal with any of that, you can just run on a treadmill. These machines are so well equipped with electronic gadgetry—heart rate monitors that automatically adjust your incline and speed to keep you in the right zone—that many runners use them even when it's nice out.

There is no question that runners have wised up since the boom days of the 1970s and 1980s. Although the early running boom put most runners on paved streets and sidewalks and left many of them with swollen joints, the sustained interest in running has led to increasing opportunities for those who prefer the soft surfaces of grass and dirt trails. Most areas have trail-running clubs these days and many cities are following the lead of Portland, Eugene, and San Francisco and maintaining dirt running trails in their city parks. An increasing number of "road" races these days actually take place on trails through the woods. Also, the boom in mountain biking has led to vast networks of trails all over the country that are ideal for running.

What's more, thirty years of research into running has helped coaches and running enthusiasts develop more effective methods for training. Although researchers have always believed that runners' performances will drop off no matter how hard they train or refine their workouts, a lot of older runners are striding across the beach to kick sand in their faces. Look at Carlos Lopes, the thirty-seven-year-old who set a world record in the marathon (26.2 miles) in 1984 when he ran 2:07. Or check out New Zealander Derek Turnbull, who broke 5 minutes for the mile and 35 minutes for the 10-kilometer at the ripe old age of sixty-five.

Most runners slow down because their maximal aerobic capacity (VO_2 max) declines. That decline probably stems from the fact that a person's MHR drops with age no matter how much he or she exercises. Many runners also can't move air in and out of their lungs as fast when they get older, and many tend to lose lean body mass—up to 4 pounds a decade after their thirty-fifth birthday—despite a diligent running program. Their leg muscles also tend to tighten and become less supple, and that shortens their stride and forces them to expend more energy than they used to with each step. All this adds up to slower times and prompts some athletes to abandon running altogether.

But there is no need to. Although beginner runners tend to get injured more often than veteran runners, most of those injuries stem from inexperience—the runner tried to do too much too soon or didn't budget enough rest or cross-training into his or her workouts. The threat of injuries shouldn't discourage you from taking up running but it should convince you to approach the sport with caution. Blend large doses of walking into your running at first, slowly whittling down those walking segments as you become more fit. And always look for opportunities to run on grass or even dirt trails—golf courses at dusk are a great place to run, as are large city parks.

Keep in mind that many runners have offset the effects of aging, and some have actually improved their aerobic capacity—and speed— as they've aged. Successful runners do this by making the best use of what they've got. Although VO_2 max declines with one's MHR, studies show that a good athlete's efficiency—the percentage of VO_2 max that he or she can use—tends to go up. A recent study of older runners, average age sixty-three, found that although they had less muscle mass, lower VO_2 maxes, and less power than a group of younger runners with similar 10-kilometer times and training schedules, the older runners had 31 percent more oxidative enzyme activity. They were able to process oxygen and remove lactic acid more efficiently, a skill they'd developed over years of training.

Getting Started

If you are a fit walker and are thinking about adding a little running to your repertoire, chances are you're making a smart decision. The interesting thing about walking and running is that fit people walking at a fast pace feel like the effort is harder than when they are jogging at the same speed. That's because walking uses fewer muscles than running, and those muscles become fatigued faster. Ironically, although jogging feels easier at those speeds, you are usually burning more calories when you jog 3 miles than when you walk them. And what's more, you burn more fat jogging those 3 miles than when walking. Of course, this is true for fit people who have to walk at a high speed to create an aerobic effort; older people who are unfit and carrying around extra weight should continue walking and monitoring their heart rates until they reach a point at which their walking has to be very fast to get their heart thumping. Then it's time to try jogging.

That doesn't mean you have to give up walking altogether. In fact, an increasing number of formal running programs around the country are based on a training and racing format that includes generous amounts of walking. Entries into the country's biggest marathon events are increasing each year, and many race organizers credit runners who walk all or part of the 26.2-mile course. Walking breaks are interspersed with running, and for many people this makes a marathon possible at a time in their lives when families and jobs don't give them enough time to train for a full-blown run at the marathon distance.

The run–walk strategy was developed by former Olympic marathoner Jeff Galloway, who himself operates training groups in forty U.S. cities. Galloway shrugs at the purists who complain that walking runners steal from the mystique of the marathon. "We're not trying to make people Olympic athletes," he says. "In a society in which 55 percent of the people are overweight, what do you want to promote?"

Training Programs

If you have been running for a while, you might be interested in adding some variety to your workouts. If you are running the same 4-mile loop from your local YMCA every day, consider branching out—adding some fast running, varied terrain, or both will dramatically improve your fitness and may rejuvenate your interest in the sport. But always be careful to add additional work in slow, steady doses; too much too soon could leave you injured.

ADDING SPEED TO YOUR WORKOUTS

If you've been running for a while and have become comfortable doing hard workouts such as tempo runs or cruise intervals, it might be time to try some speed work. This kind of workout gets you fit and ready to race.

It's probably safe to say that most runners do their speed work at a faster pace than they should. If you're a 42-minute 10-kilometer person, it's counterproductive to go to the track once a week trying to gut out 75-second quarters. You might be learning how to tol-erate lactic acid, but you're increasing your chances of injury and your body isn't learning to burn fat at higher and higher speeds—something you need more if you're going to break 40 minutes for the 10-kilometer.

That said, running economy—as measured by the percentage of oxygen you breathe in that is actually put to work creating energy for running—is improved when you train at speeds faster than your best 5-kilometer pace. One workout recommended by running ex-

You don't need to be an Olympic-caliber athlete to have a personal training program. All a training program does is give some structure to your effort—it helps you establish goals, stay on track, and measure your improvement. This is what many people need to stay with their training when work or family pressures are threatening their workouts.

There is no perfect training program that works for every runner. That is because every runner is different—some recover faster than others, some have more slow-twitch muscle fibers than others, and some get overtrained faster than others. The secret to a good training program is to attempt to incorporate very important elements, such as hill running and speed work, while giving yourself enough time to recover and rebuild. It helps for some people to run with friends; others are better off running alone. It also helps to keep your training program fresh and entertaining. Indulge yourself—run on scenic trails, look for variety in your workouts and workout locations, and above all else, keep records. A training log allows you to experiment with your training regimen because it's easier for you to document and see where you succeeded and where you didn't.

The major components of a good, overall training program include

pert Owen Anderson is 800-meter intervals at 10 seconds per 800 faster than your 5-kilometer pace, with 4- to 6-minute recoveries. This kind of workout should be done only every other week when you are preparing for a race.

Another method for improving your aerobic capacity is by running 1,200-meter repeats at a 5-kilometer pace, with an equal amount of time for a recovery jog and walk. Another strategy is running 3-minute surges with 1–2 minutes rest.

Another way to improve your aerobic capacity is by running 3-minute repeats (around 800 meters for above-average runners) at a pace equal to your best time for 3,000 meters or 5-minute repeats (around 1,500 meters) at a pace equal to your pace for a 5-kilometer run. Recovery jogs should be as long as your interval and the total mileage should be 5 to 10 percent of your weekly total. You should do these workouts for six to eight weeks leading up to a race; don't race during this kind of tough training.

speed work, tempo running (or lactate threshold training), hills, long-distance runs, strength training, and, most importantly, rest. All of these components work together to make you a faster and more efficient runner and contribute to overall fitness by putting just the right amount of stress on all your muscular and energy-delivery systems. Each has a purpose—whether it is to improve your form, teach your body to burn fat at increasing levels of effort, or improve your ability to use oxygen. With the exception of the rest component, it isn't necessary to do each of these types of workouts every week; each comes into play at different times of the year or even different times in your life.

What's important is to fashion a training program that meets your particular needs. The secret is to experiment—push yourself, let your body recover, and keep notes on how you respond. And when in doubt, take the day off.

Power and Hills

Hill training is often overlooked, but it is the best way to improve your form and learn rhythm. Proper hill running helps lengthen your stride, and beginners find it is a good way to get used to difficult running efforts that push their heart rates into the higher regions of effort. Inexperienced runners actually have more to fear from downhill running than uphill running because it is the downhill portions that often leave them with sore quadriceps muscles the next day.

There are two recommended ways to run hills: long, continuous efforts and short, sharp assaults. Experienced runners do one or the other—or a combination of the two—at least once a week. Some runners pick a hilly course and then concentrate their efforts on the uphill sections; others do hill repeats and use the downhill sections for recovery.

Here are some other tips for running up hills:

- Adjust the length of your stride to the steepness of the hill. The steeper it is, the closer you get to baby steps. Try to keep the same turnover rhythm. Use a light ankle-flicking motion, not an explosive motion.

- Never charge up a hill and then back off to recover when you reach the crest. Leave enough on the climb to run through the crest and then press the pace on the downhill. Never let your heart rate climb more than 5 or 10 beats above your training pace on the uphill and keep it within 5 beats of training pace on the downhill.
- Use your arms in a straight forward-and-back motion and concentrate on keeping your upper body relaxed. Look ahead, not down. Lengthen your stride downhill, landing on the balls of your feet with your knees slightly bent. Use the muscles in the back of your legs to push you forward.

Lactate Threshold Runs

Your lactate threshold is the point at which you are rapidly accumulating lactic acid in your blood and muscles. That's because you are demanding more energy than your aerobic system (sugar and fat burning) can supply and your body switches over to burning primarily sugar, which produces lactic acid as a byproduct. When you approach this effort level, your body adapts by increasing its number of fat-burning enzymes in your muscles and you slowly learn to burn fat at higher and higher speeds. You don't have to be training for the Olympic trials to run like this; even everyday runners who start this type of running enjoy fast, measurable improvements in their speed, fitness levels, and overall satisfaction with the sport.

There are two basic types of lactic threshold training: tempo runs and long intervals. It's best to think of this type of training as running comfortably hard—somewhere around 90 percent of your MHR or 20–30 seconds a mile slower than your fastest pace for 3 miles. At this pace you are breathing hard but you shouldn't be hurting and your muscles shouldn't be stinging; if they are, you need to slow down.

Tempo runs are continuous efforts of about 20 or 30 minutes. If you've never trained like this before, start out with shorter intervals and build into it as you get stronger. Tempo runs—like any challenging

A GOOD TRAINING PROGRAM SHOULD INCLUDE SPEED WORK, TEMPO RUNNING, HILLS, LONG-DISTANCE RUNS, STRENGTH TRAINING, AND, MOST IMPORTANT, REST.

effort—should be preceded by a warmup of at least a mile and should be followed by a 1-mile jog. Some runners also do what's known as cruise intervals, which are runs of 1,000 yards or so at lactate threshold pace, with a recovery jog of a minute or two.

Lactate threshold runs are ideal when you are short of time—even with a mile warmup and cool down, you can be finished in less than 45 minutes. You can even do them on a treadmill. Next time you can't get away from the office and have to work out on the company exercise room treadmill, try measuring your lactate threshold intervals by calories. After warming up for 100 calories, run hard for 75 calories then easy for 25 calories and repeat until you've burned up your caloric goal. You'll be surprised how fast the time goes by.

Rest and Recovery

Most successful—and healthy—runners train by the hard–easy system, which was developed by University of Oregon coaches Bill Delinger and Bill Bowerman after they noticed that their runners progressed faster when their workouts varied by intensity and duration from day

TAPERING: WHEN REST MEANS SPEED

If you have been training hard and are planning to do a race so that you can gauge your improvement, it's a good idea to alter your workout schedule in the week or weeks leading up the race. This is called tapering, and research shows it can improve performance dramatically.

In two separate studies in recent years, runners who cut their training mileage by as much as 90 percent in the week before a race and ran a decreasing number of intervals during that week

all experienced tremendous improvements in their times. After an easy warmup they did their intervals—in one case they were 400-meter intervals and in the other study runners did 500 meters—at a pace equal to their best mile times or 5-kilometer times. In the study at MacMaster University in Ontario, Canada, the runners started with five intervals and decreased the number by one each day, with none the day before the race. Their times improved by 22 percent. In the second study, runners' 5-

to day. Their system reinforced what scientists later labeled the overload and progression principle, and now many runners follow difficult workouts with 1 or 2 days of easier efforts that allow the body to replenish fuel and repair muscle. If this is done correctly, the muscle learns to repair itself faster and take on even more stress afterward. The hard–easy system cuts down on injuries but also keeps a runner's mind fresh; she can look forward to a well-earned easy day and be mentally fresh and confident to face the challenge of the next hard workout.

The hard–easy system doesn't have any hard-and-fast rules, however, and each runner has to make adjustments to fit his or her particular needs. Sometimes hard days must be followed by 2 easy days and some runners choose to do back-to-back hard days that are followed by 2 or 3 easy days. Age is also a factor, because many researchers believe older people don't recover as quickly as younger athletes do.

The overall goal, however, is to get in 2 or 3 hard days a week. Some runners, rather than trying to carve 3 hard days into a convenient 7-day training week, create a 10-day training period in order to get all the hard training and recovery running in. This makes more sense for

kilometer times improved by a stunning 29 seconds. And these were elite runners, so their times were already pretty quick. This research blew out of the water earlier principles of tapering, which called for lower mileage but slow running.

If you are tapering for a marathon or half marathon, you need to start your taper sooner. Marathoners should taper for four weeks, decreasing mileage each week by going to 75 percent of their average mileage to 50 percent to 30 percent to 15 percent the week before the race. Half-marathoners should go to 50 percent two weeks before a race to 15 percent the week before. Maintain your speed work, but cut back on the easy miles. In the last week, emphasize 5-kilometer and race-pace intervals.

The taper allows your muscles to recover while improving your glycogen stores, increasing your aerobic enzymes, and giving you a sharp, enthusiastic mental outlook. It really works.

older runners, but it requires a lot more careful planning and something of a flexible schedule. Most runners prefer to keep their long runs for Sunday morning, for instance, or their track workouts on Wednesday because they know that's a good day to sneak away from work for 2 hours.

What constitutes a hard day? This is anything that is more than 20 percent of your weekly mileage or 10 percent of your weekly mileage if it is done in the form of a speed workout. Any run longer than 30 percent of weekly total is also a hard day, and should be followed by 2 easy days.

So what's an easy day? This is anything that's less than 10 percent of weekly mileage, done at an easy pace—60 or 70 percent of your MHR or a run done at a conversational pace. Many runners take the day off or use their easy days to cross-train in the pool or on a bike, but many coaches feel it's important to run at least a little bit to promote circulation and stimulate tissue to repair itself. Try to avoid increasing your weekly mileage by adding to easy days; always increase your mileage on your hard days first; only after your body has adjusted to this new stress level should you consider increasing your easy day.

How much rest do you need? This varies from runner to runner, but for runners around age fifty, here are some general rules:

- High-mileage runs should be followed by 2 or 3 easy-mileage days (1 day can be of average length or intensity).
- High-stress or high-intensity days (speed work, tempo runs, or hills) should be followed by 2–4 easy-mileage days.
- Races should be followed by an easy day for every hard mile you ran. For instance, a hard half-marathon should be followed by roughly two weeks of easy running (with a couple of hard days allowed after you're feeling stronger).

Keeping a detailed training log is the best way to develop patterns that work best for you. You may find that you can follow a hard speed session with only 1 easy day before you're ready for your long run, or you may find you need 2 easy days. Be patient and take notes. What were your rest, training, and posttraining heart rates? Did your legs feel fresh or sluggish? Did you have enough energy?

The Long Run

Weekly long runs are a staple of almost every running program. The long, slow run is the best way to develop your cardiovascular system, but you should be very cautious about how much distance you add to your long days. Your long run should never be more than 30 percent of your weekly total, and you should never add more than 2 miles to it from one week to the next. You can safely do a long run once a week until you get up to 10 miles, at which point you should run it every two weeks. When you pass 18 miles, do your long run every third week.

Runners who are having trouble getting through their long runs or recovering quickly enough are probably running too fast. Try walking portions of it. Even experienced runners should consider walking 1 minute for every 5 minutes of running. The other thing you should do is slow down. Marathoner Jeff Galloway says the difference between feeling good after a 12-mile run and feeling poorly can be as little as 15 seconds per mile. As a rule, run 2 minutes slower on your long runs than you normally do.

Long runs are a great way to build mental strength, try out different training routes, or get together with other friends. You should always run at an easy, conversational pace, and it's always important to bring water and high-energy snacks.

Strength

Strength training is particularly important to runners as they get older because they tend to lose lean muscle mass. Those who do work out with weights tend to maintain their lean muscle mass, and those who do strength training on their legs don't get injured as much.

For your legs, exercise physiologist Owen Anderson recommends doing strides on a flat grassy area in your bare feet. Also recommended are squats, leg presses, leg curls, heel raises, toe raises, and bench step-ups. Anderson recommends that you do this kind of strength work twice a week.

Here are some general guidelines for upper-body weight training:

- Begin with a thorough warmup, including 10–15 minutes of jogging, walking, or cycling.

- Work from the larger muscle groups to the smaller groups. For instance, do bench presses, lateral pull-downs, squats, and leg presses (for muscle groups that cross two joints) first, followed by bilateral bicep curls, knee extensions, and leg curls using both legs.
- Perform one to three sets of 8 to 12 repetitions each. Choose a weight in which the last 2 or 4 repetitions are difficult. When you've worked up to 12 reps and the last ones aren't tough anymore, add weight.
- Take 1 second to do the primary movement (pulling the weight down or pushing it up) and 3 seconds to bring it back. This is where the strength comes from.
- Always cool down and stretch.

TRICKS TO AVOID POSTRUN MUSCLE ACHES

Many runners finish their first marathon and they are amazed how good they feel. They're tired, but nothing hurts and they wonder out loud whether they should have run a little harder.

The next day they are walking downstairs backwards and generally moving around like hundred-year-old bricklayers who just fell off the second story.

These folks are suffering from delayed onset muscle soreness (DOMS), a short-lived but extremely painful condition they could have avoided with the right kind of training.

Two types of exercise put this particular stress on a conditioned athlete: eccentric exercise such as downhill running, which requires the muscle to contract as it is lengthening; and exhaustive exercise, which completely drains working muscles of all glycogen.

The soreness is a result of structural and chemical damage to the cell walls of the muscle fibers, tendons, and fascia, which is the connective tissue that binds them together. Chemical substances within the tissues spill out and cause swelling that stimulates nerve ends, which send out a steady signal, sort of like the siren on an ambulance. The soreness usually doesn't kick in for 24 hours, although sometimes it's delayed for 3 days.

The best way to treat the soreness is with a little hair of the dog that bit you: Go out for an easy run. This inspires the muscle to pump out the chemical wastes.

A Better Way to Stretch

You still see runners who spread their legs, bend at the waist, and start bouncing up and down over their knees. They are stretching, they say.

What they are really doing is yanking and, in some cases, tearing their muscles. It's called ballistic stretching and if the name conjures up images of warfare and destruction, then so be it. Although ballistic stretching was popular for decades, we've come a long way in recent years and we've learned some far more effective ways to keep your muscles supple.

Stretching not only helps prevent injuries, but it can improve performance and help you maintain balance and peace of mind. Your workout may be a thumping, clenched period of tough exertion, but it

Athletes can also take some ibuprofen or aspirin. Studies have shown that icing your sore spots doesn't do much good.

Better yet, avoid the pain altogether by carbo-loading before the race and incorporating some downhill running into your workouts.

After a 2-mile warmup and some stretching, run 4 to 8 repeats down a 200- or 400-meter hill (not too steep!) at about three-quarters effort. Jog easily back to the top after each repeat and finish off with another 2-mile jog and some stretching. Do this every three weeks or so, slowly increasing your effort level. Never go full-blast—that can leave you injured—but work hard. Expect to get a little sore after each effort, but rest assured that you will come back stronger—it's the principle of overload and progression. Although one study found that just one of these sessions could reduce or prevent soreness for up to ten weeks, the experts recommend that you do a few of them over a period of several weeks to fully prepare yourself for race day.

Also plan to do some slow runs that take longer—from 30 minutes to an hour—than your expected finish time for the marathon. Remember, distance isn't important. Time is. Do these runs only every three or four weeks, with the last one at least a full month before your marathon race.

should always be followed by a quiet period where you coax new length and elasticity out of the cords that give you strength.

Stretching is particularly important as we get older. As we age, we lose some water in our cells and this makes us stiffer and less supple. Exercise counters some of that effect, but exercise combined with stretching is the best strategy to forestall those changes.

One of the effects of exercise is to shorten a muscle. When you work a muscle, you lengthen it and then contract it, and the result is a tighter bundle of fibers. But this is one training effect you don't need. A longer, more elastic muscle does work more efficiently and can be pulled farther during exercise before tiny tears are made. Runners who can maintain the frequency of their leg turnover but add an inch to the length of their stride can carve 30 seconds off their times for a 10-kilometer run. Those who can add 2 inches will take a minute off.

A longer muscle also reduces the stress on your tendons, which attach muscles to bones. Whereas a muscle can stretch to 130 percent of its resting length, a tendon can only go 4 percent. And you don't want to push them past that point; tears in tendons don't heal as quickly as muscle tears. And loose tendons and ligaments don't work as well as taut ones and can cause ankle sprains and other joint instability problems.

Most people stretch their quadriceps, hamstrings, buttocks, and hip flexor muscles with static stretching, in which you lean into stretches and hold them until the discomfort goes away. It's a simple and safe technique, but the best technique is called proprioceptive neuromuscular facilitation (PNF) stretching. This method takes advantage of the muscles' and tendons' natural protective reflexes and tricks the muscle into getting longer. It also involves isometric contractions, the tightening of a muscle without any movement occurring, as when you push against a wall.

Every muscle has a stretch reflex. When the muscle is stretched past the point of comfort, the muscle spindle—a receptor in the muscle fiber—orders the muscle to contract to protect it from tearing. The spindle also jumps into action during exercise. When the muscle is contracted while running, for instance, the spindle sends out orders to the muscle group located just opposite to it (called the antagonist muscle group) to relax. When you are running up a hill, for instance, your quadriceps contract right after your foot lands and starts to push your body up against gravity. While this is happening, the spindle is telling the hamstring to relax. This is called reciprocal innervation. The tendon also has a protective receptor known as the Golgi tendon organ (GTO); when a tendon is pulled dangerously taut, it sends a message to the muscle to relax.

PNF tricks all these mechanisms into helping you become more limber. The technique is to put the muscle into a mild stretch (similar to the easy stretch portion of the static stretch), hold it for 10 seconds, and then contract the muscle being stretched isometrically for 3–6 seconds before relaxing the muscle again and pulling it deeper into the stretch for 20–30 seconds. The isometric contraction halfway through the stretch triggers the signal from the GTO and allows the muscle to stretch out even further.

USE PNF STRETCHING TO BECOME MORE LIMBER.

An advanced form of PNF stretching takes the trickery another step further. After you begin the third step—the second, deeper stretch— you isometrically contract the muscles opposite the muscle being stretched. This takes advantage of that reciprocal innervation reflex: The spindle in the contracting muscle sends a signal out to the muscle being stretched and tells it to relax. Voilà! Your stretched muscle starts to get longer and you begin making some permanent gains in flexibility and suppleness.

Here are the four main PNF stretches runners need to know:

- **Hamstring stretch:** Sit on the ground with one leg out in front of you, toes up, knee straight. Bend the other leg at the knee and bring the sole of your foot up to the thigh of the straight leg. Lean over the straight leg until you feel slight discomfort. Hold it there 10–20 seconds. Then contract the hamstring by pressing the heel of your straight leg into the ground. Hold that for up to 6 seconds, then relax and move deeper into your stretch. You can hold that, or you can take it a step further and contract your quad, straightening your leg even more. Hold that for 30 seconds, slowly building up to 2 minutes. Repeat with the other leg.

- **Quad stretch:** Stand on one leg and bend your other leg to bring your foot back to where you can grab your ankle. Pull it toward your buttocks until you feel some discomfort. Hold it for up to 20 seconds, then contract the quad as if you are going to put your foot back down. Hold that for 3–6 seconds, then relax and pull your foot back further. Hold that for 30 seconds and work it up to 2 minutes. Take it a step further by contracting your hamstrings while you are pulling back the second time. Repeat with the other leg.

- **Buttocks stretch:** Lie on your back with one leg straight out in front, toes up, and the other bent and raised, its foot flat on the ground. Grab the bent leg behind the knee and gently pull the knee toward your chest until you feel some slight discomfort. Hold it for 20–30 seconds, then press your bent leg against your hands, as if you are trying to stretch it out. Hold that for 3–6 seconds, then relax and pull the knee back deeper into the stretch. You can simultaneously flex your hip flexor muscles and work this part of the stretch up to 2 minutes. Repeat with the other leg.

- **Calf stretch:** Lean forward against a wall or tree, one leg stretched out straight behind you, heel on the ground. Push gently into the stretch until you feel the tightness. Hold it for up to 20 seconds, then contract the calf muscle (isometrically!) as if you are trying to stand on your toes. Hold that for 3–6 seconds, then relax and go into a deeper stretch. You can simultaneously flex your shin muscles as if you were trying to pull your feet and toes toward the sky. Hold that for 30 seconds, working up to 2 minutes.

You'll make permanent gains in muscle length only by stretching after exercise, when your muscles are thoroughly warmed up. Some runners don't stretch at all before running and many like to jog a little first, stretch, and then do a full workout. A good rule: Use simple static stretches before your workout and more involved PNF stretching after. Before a race or hard workout, however, you should warm up thoroughly and stretch thoroughly using the PNF method. Jog and do some race-pace strides to see whether all the muscles you need are limber enough.

How to Treat and Avoid Running Injuries

Most running injuries are caused by inadequate warmups, ill-fitting shoes, or overexuberant workouts, and are easily preventable. Aches and pains are not uncommon after running, and most go away. Sharp pain that lasts more than 20 or 30 minutes, however, is a clue that something is wrong. Researchers are starting to notice that an increasing number of women athletes are suffering injuries. Some researchers attribute the increasing injuries to women's physiology; they have smaller ligaments, for instance, and generally have more looseness in the joints. It's also true that sporting goods manufacturers, who have spent millions enticing women into sports and physical activity, still don't design much of their gear specifically for women. Manufacturers still don't make a track-and-field shoe specifically for women; most female lines are simply scaled-down men's shoes, even though women's feet are not shaped the same way as men's feet.

FOLLOW THE HARD-EASY SYSTEM TO CUT DOWN ON INJURIES.

Most mild aches and **pains** and mild chronic conditions can be treated with a combination of **stretching** and strength workouts. A quarter of the more serious injuries runners experience are ankle sprains. Another common acute injury is a hamstring tear, which is usually caused when you run too fast and the hamstring is overpowered by the much larger quadriceps muscle in the front of the upper leg. The hamstring must be at least 60 percent as strong as the quad.

The best method for treating hamstring injuries and ankle sprains is the RICE method—rest, ice, compression, and elevation. You can still work out—swimming or rowing is usually okay with these injuries—but don't do anything that causes pain to the leg or ankle.

But if you have chronic or sharp pain that won't go away, chances are it's one of the following injuries.

Achilles Tendinitis

This is an inflammation of the Achilles tendon, the large tendon connecting the two calf muscles to the back of the heel bone. Stressing calf muscles with too much hill or speed work will cause the tendon to tighten and become inflamed, and eventually it will develop a covering of scar tissue. You know you have this if the pain close to the heel doesn't go away. Sometimes you can hear the scar tissue scraping against the tendon when the ankle is moved.

The best thing you can do is stop running, take aspirin or ibuprofen, and ice the area several times a day until the inflammation subsides. Massaging the area in semicircles will also help. Don't expect to run for up to two months—not until you can do toe raises without pain. Surgery can be done, but the scar tissue usually grows back.

The best way to prevent this is to stretch your calves diligently. If

PICKING YOUR SPOTS: PERIODIZATION

You should restrict very hard training to a three- or four-month period in which you are preparing for some races that are important to you. Older runners should keep some speed sessions in the program all year because the sudden introduction of speed can cause injury.

For most people, though, the seasons and their own schedules dictate their periods for them. For instance, Barney and Janis Klecker, both world-class distance runners, stay at home in Minnesota to train all year round because they find that the harsh winters force them into some alternative training routines that pay off. When it gets cold and snowy, they hit the cross-country ski trails or go snowshoeing. They also run more on the treadmill and in the deep end of the pool. Winter "forces you to rest a while. And you need to do different workouts, so you get out of the grind of 70–80 miles a week," Barney Klecker says.

"We all need periods of psychological and physical recovery," says Warren Finke, a coach and advisor for runners in Oregon. "After a period of racing, there should be a period of reduced training, rest and recovery leading into another sequence of base and strength building." The off-season, which is usually wintertime, is a good time for runners to experiment with cross-training or other forms of supplemental training. Work on your cycling on a stationary bike or get into the pool for lap swimming or running. Spring will come soon.

you tend to pronate (your feet rotate inward when running), get orthotics or specialized shoes.

Chondromalacia

This is the wearing away of the cartilage under the kneecap. You know you have it when you feel pain beneath or on the sides of the kneecap. The pain is most severe on the hills, and in the worst cases you can feel cartilage rubbing against cartilage when the knee is flexed. People get it from tired or weak quadriceps muscles or a muscle imbalance between weak quads and tighter hamstrings, which can pull the kneecap out of its proper alignment.

Naturally, you should stop running, ice the knee for 15 minutes two or three times a day, and take aspirin, which can block further breakdown of cartilage. Once the pain and swelling are gone, strengthen quadriceps by doing step-downs: Stand on a step or box at least 4 inches high. Keep your right quadriceps tight while you lower the left leg slowly toward the floor. Then raise it back up to the box, and relax. Repeat 40 times with each leg. Continue increasing repetitions in increments of 5 every 2 days, all the way up to 60 reps. Always stretch your quadriceps and hamstrings, and when you start running again, try wearing a rubber sleeve with a hole that fits over the kneecap, which can help the knee track better.

Iliotibial Band Syndrome

This is inflammation and pain on the outside of the knee, where a ligament that runs along the outside of the thigh is rubbing against the femur. You feel a dull ache a mile or two into a run that lingers during the run but disappears soon after you stop. In severe cases, the pain can be sharp, and the outside of the knee can be tender or swollen.

It's caused by any number of things: bowed legs, old shoes, even a single tough workout. Most often it's caused when people step up their training too fast.

You should see a doctor or a physical therapist, who can give you some stretches to do. Also ice the knee for 15–20 minutes after running, try self-massage on the area, and stretch your hamstrings and other leg muscles. You should be back to easy running in two to four weeks.

Plantar Fasciitis

The plantar fascia is a thick, fibrous band of tissue on the bottom of the foot from the heel to the base of the toes. When it is stressed and tears, scar tissue moves in and makes the problem worse. It feels like a bone bruise and it hurts most in the morning or at the beginning of a run.

You need to take aspirin or ibuprofen daily and ice the area several times a day. A doctor or physical therapist can accelerate the healing process with ultrasound, massage, and a brace, but if that doesn't work, a doctor may recommend surgery. It helps to stretch your calf muscles and to strengthen your foot muscles by picking up marbles or golf balls with your toes. While you have the golf ball out, roll your foot over the ball from the base of each toe to the heel and back again to help stretch the fascia.

Shin Splints

These occur when the tendons on the inside of the front of the lower leg become inflamed. The pain—a throbbing sensation about halfway down the inside of the shin—is worse at the start of a run, but can go away during a run once the muscles are loosened up. You get this when your calves are tired or haven't been stretched enough or if you overpronate. Running on hard surfaces doesn't help. Some runners will run right through mild shin splints if it's early in their training, but if the problem persists, you have to take painkillers, ice the area and cut down or stop running altogether until the pain is gone. If none of that works, find a sports-minded podiatrist. He or she might prescribe some orthotics, but surgery is rarely recommended.

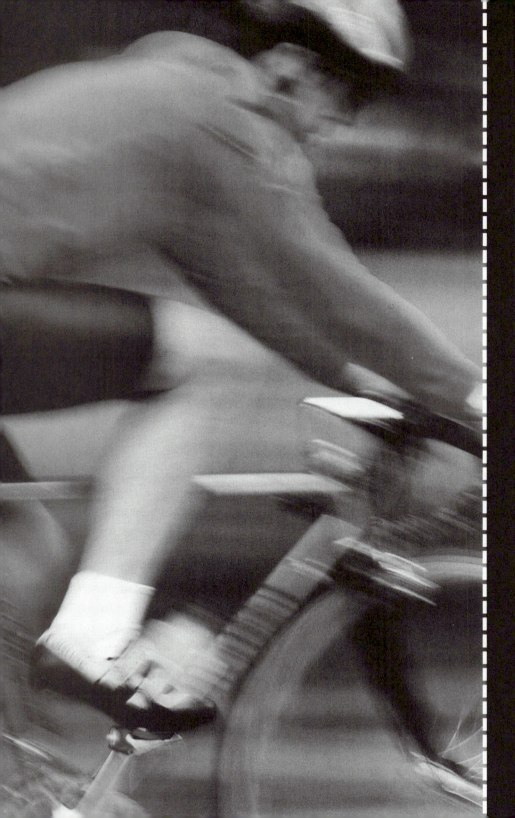

CHAPTER 8

CYCLING

Many athletes as they get older turn to cycling as a way to stay fit or improve their overall fitness. Of the nation's 57.4 million cyclists, almost 40 percent are over age forty. That's because cycling is a nonimpact activity that doesn't hammer the joints, making it easier to recover from hard workouts and easier to stay in shape if you're injured.

The advent of convenient indoor machines has made it easier to make cycling your main form of exercise. In addition to stationary bikes, with their computer panels showing how many miles you've ridden or how many calories you've burned, there is a new generation of less expensive but more challenging spinning stationary bikes, which more closely replicate actual road riding and have spawned increasingly popular spinning classes at health clubs across the country. These classes give you all the motivation of a good group ride without the threat of crashes or the inconvenience of a flat tire. Although most avid riders once considered indoor riding the unfortunate price to pay for staying in shape during the winter, many now make indoor riding a vital part of their overall fitness and training plan.

OF AMERICA'S 57.4 MILLION CYCLISTS, 40 PERCENT ARE OVER FORTY.

Cycling is one of the sports recommended by the American College of Sports Medicine for a general fitness program because it uses a large group of muscles and most people know how to do it. It's not hard to reach aerobic levels of training on a bicycle, and a growing number of bike trails and designated bike routes has made it easier for many of us to incorporate riding into our regular routines.

What's more, cycling is a great sport to carry on late in life. If you stopped exercising for a while and put on some extra weight, you should consider cycling as a way of dropping that weight. The reason for that is that cycling allows you to burn fat while riding—if the effort is hard enough—but also teaches your body to burn fat afterward as you refuel your spent energy supplies. Also, that extra weight you're carrying around could lead to injuries if you were a runner—it magnifies the pounding your joints take—but it isn't as much of a factor on a bike.

Although many cyclists find that they lose their raw power and sprinting speeds as they age, most cyclists are able to hold onto their endurance. Take Mario Bau, for instance. He rode professionally in the

Tour of Italy in the 1950s, and today, at age sixty-five, still logs 200 miles a week on his bike. The long rides in the hills outside his home in Pasadena, California, he says, "are still easy."

"You no longer have the power of a person in their twenties, but you do keep your endurance," Bau says.

In fact, one study has shown that cyclists have been able to maintain their aerobic capacity for ten years beyond their peak periods of competitive cycling. Perhaps the best example of this is Ned Overend. Six years after winning the world mountain biking title, Overend competed in the 1996 Summer Olympic Games mountain bike race in Atlanta at age forty-one. That's good for those of us who like to ride for fitness but have no aspirations of making the Olympics—it means we can still use the sport to maintain our aerobic fitness after an age when most people are slowly losing theirs.

If you're turning to cycling as a cross-training exercise or to give your battered legs a break from running, keep in mind that your MHR tends to be lower during cycling than during running. The experts aren't sure why, but one theory is that blood seems to stay longer in the legs during cycling, reducing the amount of blood pushed back into the heart and thus reducing the volume squeezed back out. If your MHR is 178 for running, for instance, it might be only 171 for cycling. Standing up out of the saddle might increase your heart rate without any increase in speed or apparent effort, and putting your hands down on the drops will lower your heart rate when you're riding on a stationary bike.

To get the most out of cycling, many riders break their training into five distinct zones based on effort level: easy riding for active recovery, endurance riding to improve aerobic capacity, lactate threshold to improve your fat-burning abilities at high effort levels, aerobic capacity training to improve efficiency, and anaerobic training to improve sprinting. Most of us will find that the first three zones give us all we need to stay fit and to make the most of the short amount of time we have for exercise. But be forewarned: If you ever get daring and decide to ride with the beginners at the next Tuesday night citizen's race, you might catch the racing bug and decide to start training in all five zones.

You'll find that bike racing runs the gamut of physiological demands—

from the blistering anaerobic stress of a 45-minute time trial or criterium to the voluminous energy and oxygen demands of a 6-hour century ride—and your training will be dictated by these demands.

Here's a rundown of the five zones and how much time you should spend in each:

- **Active recovery:** Use this after long rides or hard hilly rides that bring your heart rate up into the 80 to 90 percent region. This easy riding of 1–2 hours is a good way to flush waste products from your system and get some fresh blood and oxygen deep into your capillaries and muscles.
- **Endurance training:** This is the best zone for overall fitness and fat-burning, and should make up most of your riding time. Pick a course that has rolling hills but no extended climbs or descents. If your MHR on a bike is about 170 beats per minute, this zone is in the 122–145 beats per minute range. Try to stay in the lower end of this range, however; go too hard and you start putting some moderate stress on your system and you need to budget in some recovery time. Riders tend to spend too much time in the high end of this range and not enough in the lower end.
- **Lactate threshold:** This is for more serious riders, but even low-key cyclists will enjoy blending these rides into their training from time

RULES OF THE TRAIL

Although bikes have undergone some dramatic technological changes over the decades, none is as dramatic as the evolution of the mountain bike. It started in the early 1970s in Northern California when a group of friends started racing old bikes with balloon tires on Mount Tamalpais, but today mountain bikes make up more than 60 percent of the bicycle market. Those old clunkers of the 1970s have been replaced with $4,000-dollar models complete with shocks fore and aft, extruded aluminum and titanium frames, thermoplastic wheels, and disc brakes.

These bikes resurrected a moribund industry and put hundreds of thousands of people into the backcountry, where they have come face-to-face with hikers and horseback riders, and not always with an exchange of friendly greetings. Such has been the growth of mountain biking that it's not unusual for the bikes to be banned from certain trails, and trails where they

to time. There are basically two types of workouts: cruise intervals and tempo rides. Cruise intervals are repeats of 5–12 minutes in length at 85 to 90 percent of your MHR. You do three to five of these intervals with rests of 2 or 3 minutes. Really fit cyclists will go up to 20 minutes on a cruise interval, resting for 5 or 6 minutes. Steady inclines are a good place to get your heart rate up for these and improve your strength and efficiency. Tempo riding is an extended effort of up to 40 minutes. Citizen races are a good place to get these workouts in as long as you don't get carried away and start racing at your maximum level.

- **Aerobic capacity:** This is the really tough stuff, the upper 160s of your heart rate. You're still doing intervals here, but shorter ones, 2 to 5 minutes long. You'll do three to five of them. Recover for the same amount of time that you rode hard. Again, hills are a good place to achieve the heart rate you're looking for. This kind of training really isn't necessary for fitness cyclists, but if you race at all, even with beginners, you'll need this gear to bridge from one pace group to the next one up or to answer another rider's breakaway move. Or make a move of your own.

- **Anaerobic capacity:** This gives you the speed and energy you need for the finish. Sometimes a 120-mile race boils down to the last

are allowed are often posted with signs urging cyclists avoid tearing up trails with ruts that promote erosion.

Here are some rules to keep in mind if you hit the trail on your bike:

- Ride on open trails only. Don't trespass, and honor road or trail closure signs. Stay out of federal and state wilderness areas.
- Practice low-impact cycling. Cancel the ride if the soil is too soft, such as after a rain, and your riding might tear up the trail. Don't create new trails.
- Control your bike and stay alert.
- Always yield the trail. Make your approach known well in advance (a bell works well for this) and always slow down to a walking pace when passing someone.
- Take directions from horseback riders before passing them.
- Be self-sufficient at all times. Carry extra water, food, and equipment.

30 seconds and the riders who have done sprint training well are the ones who win. These are short sprints of up to 15 seconds at your absolute maximum effort. You're doing three sets of up to five sprints in each set, with a minute of rest between each sprint and up to 5 minutes between each set. You're working on explosive power and bike handling here, too, in addition to learning how to produce massive quantities of lactic acid.

Getting Started

Although many cyclists do some staggering training—300 miles a week isn't uncommon among elite riders—most good riders can get by on a lot less. Ned Overend, for example, trains as little as 10 or 11 hours a week, but he makes sure that his rides have purpose and aren't longer than they need to be.

Any kind of serious cycling training that involves hard intervals shouldn't come before you've put down a good base of training. For most riders, this means at least 500 miles of relaxed riding over several weeks. Many riders spend up to twelve weeks building a base with a lot of easy riding and spinning.

If riding is your primary form of exercise, research has shown that riding just once or twice a week isn't enough to develop or maintain good fitness. You'll need to do at least four rides a week, although each ride doesn't have to be a 100-miler. One study showed that cyclists who go from three rides to four rides a week see a big boost in their fitness levels.

A successful fitness program for cycling includes the following ingredients:

- Seven to 10 hours a week of training on the bike. Keep in mind that bikes are the most efficient form of vehicle ever invented, so you have to concentrate to make it a workout. You have to spend more time on a bike than you do running to get the same effect, so keep that in mind when you're budgeting time for exercise.
- Two high-quality workouts a week, such as hill climbs or time trials—timed rides over a set course, preferably one that doesn't have a lot of traffic lights and other interruptions.

- One long ride a week, always followed by an easy, short-mileage day. Many experts recommend that your long day be equal to the length of your longest race, but if you aren't interested in racing, think of the long day this way: You want to finish the ride tired, but not so entirely spent that you couldn't hop back on the bike and ride another 10 miles. Try to leave a little gas in the tank. These long rides not only trigger the physiological adaptations you need for greater endurance, but also get you used to spending a long time in the saddle. The all-important recovery rides you do the next day should be at no more than 50 to 60 percent of your MHR.

TO PREVENT INJURIES, ALWAYS RIDE WITHIN YOUR SKILL LEVEL.

- Weight training. In 1997, Australian cyclist Anna Wilson became one of the few women to ride 45 kilometers (28 miles) in an hour, and a big part of her training was the strength workouts she did in the gym each week. Her success raised questions about a study of female cyclists that showed strength training did little to improve their power output. Even though the jury is still out on weight training for female cyclists, weight training is still a widely accepted way for older athletes to match the power of younger riders. A study at the University of Maryland showed that cyclists could ride at submaximal tempo with less effort after training with weights. Work your upper body and your lower body, and if you don't have access to a weight room, do push-ups and pull-ups. If you can get to the gym, consider a wide range of exercises, from squats and leg presses to bench presses, heel raises, leg curls, and dead lifts.

- Regular stretching. Tina Renteria, a forty-five-year-old cyclist who has ridden the length of the United States twice, credits stretching with keeping her injury-free over the years. Make sure to stretch the quadriceps, but don't neglect the hamstrings.

- Overload training. As in any sport, you will continue to improve if you continue to stress your body. That means periodically making your intervals a little faster, your hills a little steeper, your long ride a little longer.

How Hills Can Improve Your Fitness

Jack Hartman was a member of the U.S. Olympic Cycling Team in Rome, competing in the track events. Today, at age fifty-seven, he spends most of his time on the road, often dominating national age-group races. The secret to his long-lasting success?

Hills.

"Hills get you fit and they help build power," Hartman says. "It involves all the elements of good cycling—shifting, weight distribution, balance, momentum, concentration, and bike handling."

Everybody knows you work harder on the hills than on the flats—an average-size rider on a lightweight road bike burns an additional 22 calories for every 100 feet of elevation gain—but that doesn't mean many cyclists use hills to their advantage. Most cyclists find it easy to come up with reasons not to attempt long, extended climbs.

Other riders thrive on hills. They enjoy finding just the right gear and cadence for the hill, and the proper mindset that allows them to keep pumping long after the brain has made its plea to quit.

BREAKING THE MONOTONY

Here are a couple of workouts to add some variety to your training:

- Interval pedaling with one leg. After warming up for at least 15 minutes, find a flat stretch and pedal for 3 minutes at 50 rpm with just one leg. The opposite leg is out of the toe clips and off to the side. When the 3 minutes is up, pedal easily with both legs for a few minutes and then do the same 3-minute, 50-rpm interval with your other leg. Do three sets for a complete workout. You can also do a speed set with 100-rpm intervals.
- Climbing high. Many riders like to do hill workouts but they do most of these rides in the saddle because that's the fastest and most efficient method. Next time try doing that long climb standing up. Drop down two cogs from your usual climbing gear and get up out of the saddle, keeping your back straight and your hips forward. The beauty of this effort is that it recruits some muscle fibers—the glutes, hamstrings, biceps, and deltoids—that normally get to rest on the climbs. Don't drop into the saddle unless you need a rest, and then sit for only 3 minutes at a time.

But climbing can be fun, and is a valuable exercise for all levels of cyclists. Beginners need to make sure they have put down a good base of training before they start tackling hills. But once they have the strength they need, hills can provide a great break from the regular routine. Hills provide great views, and with modern bikes with a multitude of gears and lightweight frames, it's possible to climb hills at a comfortable pace.

The secret to good climbing is to concentrate on pushing each pedal forward, then pulling back in a smooth stroke. Lifting and pressing pedals wastes energy, but following an 11 o'clock to 5 o'clock pattern helps. As the right crank moves toward the 11 o'clock position, pedal forward and down. Keep the pedal pressure on until the crank reaches 5 o'clock, then start pulling back and up on the pedal. Pretend you have gum on your shoe and you're trying to scrape it off.

Climbs on a mountain bike are a little trickier. Trail climbs are usually shorter, but they are often steeper and the ground conditions are more unreliable. On dirt, it's important to keep weight on the back wheel for traction while maintaining pressure on the front tire so it doesn't spin out. Getting out of the saddle on a steep dirt trail takes a lot of practice and shouldn't be attempted until you have plenty of confidence.

Eating Right

Because cyclists need to go for long rides to gain maximum aerobic fitness, it's important for riders to pay attention to their need for food and drink while exercising. One study found that when one group of cyclists rode at 90 percent of their aerobic strength and didn't drink, their performance declined within 15 minutes when compared to a similar group of cyclists who drank some water while working at the same speed. Proper hydration is particularly important for cyclists: You should drink at least 20 ounces of fluid during each training session because the wind often keeps your skin dry and you're not aware of how much you are sweating. Some riders set an alarm on their watch or handlebar computer to remind them to drink every 15 or 20 minutes.

Most riders have at one time or another experienced a bonk. This is an overwhelming sense of fatigue and hunger, and it's a sign that you've run out of glycogen to keep your aerobic fires burning. You can stave off the effects with a quick, simple snack—a piece of fruit or an energy bar—but it's better to keep the bonk at bay by eating before it arrives. Bananas, gels, crackers—many sweet, simple foods will do the trick.

Complex carbohydrate drinks can also help you on your ride. Commercial sports drinks are good but they're also expensive. Some riders mix maltodextrin, a corn starch molecule broken down into glucose polymers, with water or other drinks because it increases the energy content without adding a sugary taste. Adding a half cup of maltodextrin to a 7 percent sugar drink in a 16-ounce water bottle triples the calorie content of the drink.

Progressing into Racing

Although racing isn't nearly as popular among fitness riders as it is among casual runners, there are still opportunities for those who want to give it a try. Many riders find that racing adds an important incentive to their training, in addition to giving them a challenging workout. Always use caution, however. Pick a race that has categories so that you can ride with people who have similar abilities and fitness levels, and always stay alert when riding in a group. Although it's more dangerous than solo riding, group riding has its own special allure, particularly when you start to experience the exhilaration of drafting (riding in another rider's slipstream) and working with other riders to improve the group's overall speed.

Most coaches will tell you that the best way to get a fast time for any time trial or race is to maintain an even pace throughout. It's good advice. A number of studies on cyclists and runners have shown that starting fast or starting slow isn't going to get you there faster than trying to maintain a steady speed and rhythm. In one study, nine well-trained cyclists did a 2,000-meter time trial, completing the first 1,000 meters at a predetermined pace, including very slow, slow, even-paced, fast, and very fast, and then finishing the final 1,000 as fast as possible. The even-pacers did the best, and the slow starters were 4.3 percent slower. Anecdotal evidence backs this finding up: When researchers examined Olympic gold medal cyclist Chris Boardman during a 50-mile time trial on an undulating course, Boardman's heart rate never varied by more than 5 beats from his 178-beats-per-minute average as he raced to a win in 1:44:49. That's pretty even pacing.

If you enjoy racing, however, you don't always have the luxury of riding a steady pace. In bike races, there are often sudden breakaways to which you may need to respond, and very often these surges will push your heart rate up to its maximum limit for a time. One study compared two groups of elite cyclists who rode at different pacing strategies for 2.5 hours before doing a 20-kilometer time trial. One group rode at a steady pace and the second group varied their pace 12 percent above and below the steady pace of the other group—in other words, surging and then coasting to recover. Although each group expended identical average power measurements during their rides, the riders in the steady-pace group were more than 90 seconds faster for the 20-kilometer time trial. The important point is that you should train for the type of riding you want to do. If you aren't interested in racing but you want to get very fit and fast on a bike, remember the steady-pace strategy. If you want to improve your standing at the Tuesday night races at the reservoir, however, prepare yourself for a little uncertainty.

Mountain bike racers don't have the luxury of even pacing. Although most road racing starts are leisurely rolling starts, mountain bike racers have to sprint at the gun so they can establish good position in the group as the race funnels into a single track trail. This requires the cyclists to use anaerobic energy early on so that later in the race they don't have to expend a lot of additional aerobic energy to move past other cyclists on a narrow race course.

How to Avoid Injuries

Now that more than 25 million Americans own mountain bikes and nearly 100,000 of those people are entering organized races, doctors are starting to see an alarming increase in injuries resulting from mountain biking. The number of reported mountain bike injuries more than doubled from 1994 to 1995, when 48,000 riders suffered injuries.

Crashes have become part and parcel of off-road biking. One survey of 650 mountain bikers found that nearly 80 percent had been injured in a crash and that 20 percent of those cyclists had injuries so severe that they needed to seek medical help. Doctors are seeing an increasing number of mountain bikers with injured shoulders, clavicle fractures, and broken fingers, arms, and wrists. One encouraging note: Because most mountain bikers (an estimated 90 percent) wear helmets, only about 12 percent of those who need medical attention are diagnosed with a concussion. Severe head injuries are rare.

Most people get injured because they are riding recklessly down a hill. One study showed that nearly two-thirds of those 48,000 injuries occurred on descents when riders were going too fast for their skill levels. Competitors, pushing themselves in the heat of battle, are four times more likely to suffer severe injuries than recreational riders, and they, too, are more likely to crash on the downhill portions of the trail. The worst injuries occur when riders are pitched over their handlebars, after braking too hard with their front brakes or after striking an object. For some reason, female cross-country racers are more likely to be thrown over the handlebars than men.

The best way to prevent these traumatic injuries is to slow down and ride within your skill level. Master the fundamentals before you take off on a screaming descent through the trees. And always wear a helmet. If you're going to enter one of those kamikaze downhill sprints, make sure you wear a full facial helmet and as much shoulder, chest, and extremity padding as your dignity allows. Always check your brakes and the rest of your bike before riding, and take along a pump, spare tubes, a patch kit, and wrenches.

Mountain bikers are also subject to an array of overuse injuries. A survey of 265 riders found that 30 percent of them had recently felt some knee pain and that nearly 40 percent had lower-back pain while riding. One in five reported sore wrists and numb hands. Many of these problems can be caused by a poorly fitted bike but others result from riders pushing themselves too hard early in the season.

A lot of times cyclists with overuse injuries help heal themselves by continuing to ride—although they need to cut back on their mileage, stay away from hills, and maintain an easy, high-rpm cadence. Keep a cadence between 80 and 100 rpm. It's more efficient and it's less stressful on your knees. "When you pedal in the 40-, 50- or even 60-rpm range, it produces a fair amount of sheer force on the knee," says Dr. Edward R. Laskowski, codirector of the Sports Medicine Center at Mayo Clinic, Rochester, Minnesota. Get a bike computer with a cadence meter.

It's also important to make sure your bike fits you properly. Here are a few common problems associated with both mountain biking and road cycling and the adjustments you can make to improve them:

- **Sore neck:** Raise your handlebars or move the saddle forward so you don't have to reach as far. Also remember to move your hands around frequently and keep your arms bent at the elbows. Consider adding front suspension if you don't have it.
- **Knee pain:** This could be what's called iliotibial band friction syndrome. You need to check to make sure your knee flexes at 30–35 degrees at the bottom of the pedal stroke and that your cleats are adjusted so your toes are pointing forward or slightly to the outside.
- **Sore Achilles tendon:** Try moving your cleat back so your foot is positioned better over the pedal. If your hamstrings are also sore, try moving the saddle forward or down.
- **Lower back pain:** This usually goes away as you get in better shape, but if it's bothering you early in the season, raise your handlebars. You can lower them as the season progresses.

Proper Bike Handling

Bike handling is an important skill to develop no matter what type of bike you ride. Mountain bikers often spend at least 1 day a week working just on technique, for both climbing and descending. Proper braking, lofting (jerking up on the handlebars to get the front tire over a rock or stump), and balancing back over the rear tire to keep from tumbling on a steep descent are all essential to the sport.

Road cyclists need to develop some skills, too. The best road cycling is found in group rides, whether in a citizens' race or a training ride with some friends, and that means you'll want to learn how to draft (ride directly behind another rider), corner in groups, and keep your bike quiet (controlled) while you're sprinting your guts out in a pack. These things all take practice and shouldn't be taken for granted; you'll come to realize this fairly quickly if you clip somebody's tire at 20 miles per hour.

And you probably have a few things to learn about aerodynamics. Some riders have introduced such radical body positions—such as leaning so far over the handlebars that it looks like they are trying to touch their nose to their front tire—that their styles have been banned from use in competitions. You don't have to go that far. Just keep your arms tucked into your trunk and keep your head down. The trick is staying relaxed while maintaining your full view of the road in front of you. If you take the right precautions, it will be a long road without too many bumps.

RESISTANCE MOVEMENT: OVERCOMING AIR, GROUND, AND GRAVITY

In any kind of cycling, three forces affect speed: rolling resistance, air resistance, and gravity.

Rolling resistance isn't a big deal in road racing—those bikes are equipped with skinny, high-pressure tires with almost no tread. There's not a lot of friction there. And air resistance isn't much of an issue either because most road races are contested in large groups of riders known as pelotons. In a peloton, riders trade off riding out in front, and those behind the leaders are drafting the lead cyclists, expending significantly less energy to maintain the same speed as those in front.

The most significant force in road cycling, then, is gravity, and that's why you see pelotons break up when groups of riders encounter a sustained climb. The strongest climbers—very often these are the shortest and lightest riders—bolt to the front and break away while the heavier riders labor in the back. With equal bike-handling skills, heavier riders will move downhill faster than lighter riders, but not fast enough to make up for what they lose on the uphill climb.

The three factors affecting cycling speed play a much greater role in mountain biking. Mountain bikes have wider wheels and heavier treads than road bikes, making rolling resistance a significant force to overcome. And because drafting rarely comes into play on mountain bike rides, each rider is on her own against air resistance. But gravity is what mountain biking is all about. Mountain bike races aren't contested on flat courses, so for the most part you are either climbing or descending. And although the climbs are often very demanding, the descents are no piece of cake either. Mountain bikers are braking, negotiating, plotting courses, and shifting their body weight around to get down the hill, and this takes time and energy.

Despite these energy-sapping qualities, the mountain bike seems to be better equipped for climbing. Several studies have shown that a high cadence increases efficiency and overall speed on hills, and mountain bikes, with their tiny front sprockets and wide-ranging gear clusters, allow a high cadence. Think about how easy it is next time you're on that single track, climbing a 15 percent slope.

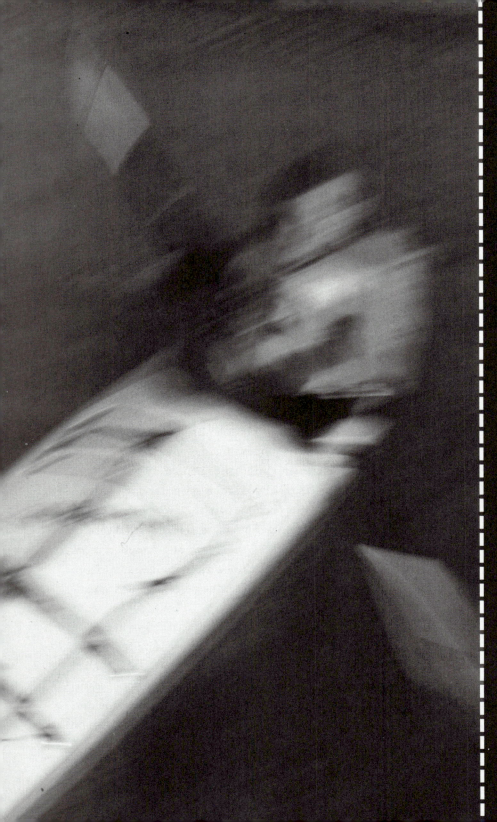

CHAPTER 9

ROWING AND PADDLE SPORTS

The coach is lean and muscled, hard from all those years in the boat. She runs a tough practice. Rowing is not about gliding, it's about strength and thrust and the laws of physics that talk about power transferred over a fulcrum. You win through the technical application of force, and you don't win by coasting. That's why the crew leaves drenched, spent, their hands and arms swollen and feeling punished.

And the day is just dawning.

It could be any crew from any college or prep school in the country. The coach could be any tough old salt who ever blew a whistle over a boat churning up the Naugatuck River or the Charles. But it isn't. This crew is a group of women approaching midlife, and their coach is a wiry woman with steel-blue eyes who teaches elementary school near Sacramento, California.

ROWING WORKS VIRTUALLY EVERY MAJOR MUSCLE GROUP.

Rowing—they called it "crew" back when we were in college—has moved beyond the quiet, dignified confines of the Ivy League and green-blue rivers of New England and has gone mainstream. A new breed of sturdy recreational shells makes it possible to row in rougher water than traditional racing shells could tolerate, and the lower price of boats has made this physically demanding and emotionally satisfying sport available to an increasing number of people.

And nowhere, it seems, is this sport more popular than among women who are approaching the challenges of their forties and fifties. That's because it's a great way to get in shape. Consider the case of Leslie Graves, who was forty-two and sedentary and weighed more than 200 pounds when her three athletic sisters convinced her to join them in training for the four-person shell for the World Masters Championship. Her sisters had all competed in crew in college—her older sister, Carie, had earned a gold medal in the women's eight in 1984—but Leslie had never competed. But with a workout plan devised by Carie, Leslie began training and not only did she learn the technical skills of rowing, she dropped 40 pounds and wasn't shy about inviting strangers to feel her biceps. "Most people would look at me and say, 'She'll give up in two weeks,'" Leslie said. "Only the sisters knew it would happen."

The Benefits of Rowing

Elite rowers train many years to develop the strength and technique they need to excel, but amateur rowers can still pick up the sport fairly quickly and gain immediate aerobic benefits from it. Many find it to be among the toughest sports they've ever attempted. Done right, rowing works virtually every major muscle group in your body, from your calves, hamstrings, and quadriceps to your back, stomach, shoulders, and arms. It's nonjarring and aerobically demanding, and although winter often puts a damper on open-water training, indoor machines are just as challenging and can help build the mental toughness you need. Indoor rowing has developed into a sport in its own right, with achievement clubs and rowing competitions on the Internet. And most good indoor rowing machines come equipped with a performance monitor, showing such things as heart rate and power generated, that you can use to gauge your progress.

People who can no longer participate in sports such as soccer or running often turn to rowing because it allows them to continue being competitive and active without further aggravating sports injuries. Done right, the rowing stroke provides little room for the serious injury often found in contact and high-impact sports.

Then, of course, there is the setting and the sensations. Few sports can match the satisfaction you feel as your shell skims across the water, thrust forward by your own power. Newcomers to the sport often describe it as addictive, and although veteran rowers aren't always so effusive, it should be noted that many have a hard time retiring from the elite ranks, despite the grueling demands and anonymity of the sport. Then there is the setting: the quiet rivers, reservoirs, and brackish bays where scullers toil in quiet determination.

In his book on rowing, *The Shell Game*, Stephen Kiesling talks of the "symphony of motion" that draws athletes to the sport of rowing.

"As dawn breaks over the river, the shell is lifted from its rack out into the morning. On another rack the oars hang ready to be greased and slipped into the locks. Then, awakened to the river and the feel of the oars, the oarsmen blend in fulfillment of the shell. The symphony is not of competition. It is the synchronous motion over water, the harmonic flexing of wood and muscle, where each piece of equipment and every oarsman is both essential to, and the limit of, motion itself."

Getting Started

Let's face it: Most of us, no matter how intrigued we are by the sport of rowing, aren't going to go out and buy a $2,000 shell and start rowing. But if you have been down to the marina, seen the teams training, and want to give it a go, look into classes you can take or clinics you can sign up for. Even if you've been training on an ergometer at the health club, chances are good you'll need some coaching to improve your stroke. Remember, it is more important to learn proper technique than it is to develop a set of back muscles that knot up like a weightlifter with each stroke. Good technique will eventually bring on the muscles, but heavy muscles won't correct poor technique—in fact, they sometimes stand in the way of it.

That said, it will pay off to be in pretty good shape before you even get in the boat. Although the best way to get in shape for rowing is by rowing, it could be discouraging to finally get in the boat and burn out after just a few minutes. So try to get into good cardiovascular shape before even attempting to crew. It also wouldn't hurt to hit the weights a little bit. No matter how fit you think you are, rowing has a way of making even the best athletes feel weak and winded. Be prepared for that. There is a reason why rowing produces some of the best athletes in the world, and that's because it is a very demanding sport.

And it helps to keep in mind that good rowing is as much physics as it is physiology. You have fulcrums and force–time curves and arc areas and fat middles. It is a very technical sport, a very complex uncoiling of kinetic energy. Your body adapts to the demand of the sport by developing the muscles, enzymes, capillaries, and energy delivery systems it needs to make you an efficient rower, and it makes these adaptations over a broad spectrum of muscle fibers and neural pathways. The problem for rowers comes, as it does for swimmers, when your technique is off somewhat—you are less efficient than you could be, and you drop your oar in too soon or fail to maintain a steady pull through the stroke. If you keep rowing that way, your neuromuscular system becomes hard-wired to perform that way and you develop habits that are difficult and painful to break. You can practice a better stroke, but if you don't concentrate, you'll fall back into your old way of doing things because that's what your body is used to.

THE
CHARACTER-
ISTICS OF A
GOOD
ROWER

149

Changing your stroke—even a little bit—can quickly become exhausting. And when you become exhausted, you fall back into what your body is accustomed to doing: rowing the wrong way. That is why you see teams of elite rowers going through hour after hour of painstaking drills designed to break down each component of their stroke to emphasize just the right motor units you want recruited in the effort.

The Characteristics of a Good Rower

Although international rowing competition is split into two weight classes—lightweight and open—the best rowers tend to be big. Because the faster rowers are those who have high stroke power and a long stroke length, the sport tends to favor tall, lean rowers with long arms and a tall sitting height. A study of elite heavyweight rowers showed the men were an average of 6-feet-3 and 194 pounds and the women were 5-feet-11, 169 pounds. That's a lot of beef being hauled around on those tiny boats. These dimensions have stayed about the same for more than three decades, although the study showed rowers have less body fat today than their counterparts in the 1960s. The best rowers of the lightweight class (under 157.5 pounds for men and under 129.8 pounds for women) have even less body fat—5 to 7 percent for men and under 15 percent for women.

Rowing builds some very fine athletes. When the maximal oxygen consumption at the height of intense exercise for male rowers is measured, their aerobic capacity is roughly 1.75 times higher than that of sedentary men of the same age. And their aerobic capacity is only 8 percent or so behind the measurements for the world's best cross-country skiers, who are often considered to be the best-trained athletes in the world.

Although they lag behind skiers in aerobic capacity, rowers tend to have the biggest hearts of all endurance athletes. Cross-country skiers, water polo players, and cyclists aren't far behind. In addition to their big pumps, rowers also can have thicker heart walls, a characteristic more often linked to hypertension. It's nothing to be worried about, though; it's an adaptation the heart makes to unusual demands rowing puts on it. Not only is the muscle expanding and getting stronger so it can deliver oxygen to working muscles, but the mechanics of rowing puts pressure on the wall and the muscle responds the same way a bicep would: it gets thicker. Studies have shown that the heart wall thins out when heavy training diminishes.

Good rowers seem to have an abundance of slow-twitch muscle fibers, and those fibers are laced with an intricate network of capillaries and mitochondria—just what you expect in a well-trained athlete. One curiosity: Rowers' individual muscle fibers tend to be thicker than those of other endurance athletes. Normally the fibers adapt with small diameters, which aids the movement of oxygen, but rowers are different because the demands of their sport are different. The stroke frequency of rowing is much lower than the repetitions for cycling and running, but the amount of force that must be produced is much higher for each rep, leading to the thicker cords. Another thing that sets rowers apart is their ability to generate power with both legs simultaneously. Those who don't row can generate only about 80 percent of the power they can produce with each leg working alone. Rowers learn to narrow that gap considerably.

The best rowers also have a tremendous lung capacity. Their respiratory muscles are not only helping push oxygen out to hard-working muscles, they are also contracting to help generate force for the stroke. Another advantage of rowing is that it seems to develop denser bones in the spine, arms, and pelvis bone, all sensitive areas for those who are prone to osteoporosis.

The Technique of Rowing

The best rowers are as graceful as they are mechanical. They curl up like a loaded spring and then burst forth in a flurried sequence of levers, pulleys, and fulcrums, throwing their legs, arms, backs, and stomachs into a controlled explosion of strength and propulsion. Rowing falls into the same category as swimming and climbing—self-propulsion sports that don't involve running. As in those sports, finding the right rhythm and central point of power takes hours of practice and training. Tiff Wood, the great American sculler and a member of the 1984 Olympic team, once figured he exercised 600 hours a year, with almost 500 of those hours spent with hands on the oars. But during that year he might race a total of 130 minutes at most. Four-time Olympic gold medalist Steven Redgrave works out about 42 hours a week for about an hour of racing a year. Few sports require so much of their athletes.

Scullers begin their stroke by bending their knees, sliding forward in their seats, and stretching their arms out in front of them fully extended. The legs move first, thrusting the seat back as the oar blades slip into the water, a moment known as the catch. As the butt and leg muscles extend the legs out, the back muscles methodically bring the torso to an erect position and the arms begin to pull. The biceps pull the oar handles forward, signaling the upper back and latissimus dorsi muscles into action as well. Finally the rower's elbows collapse, the blades emerge from the water and the boat suddenly seems to stream forward, as if it has caught a sudden tailwind. The rower then engages her hamstring muscles to pull the seat forward to start another stroke.

Racing singles are often only about 12 inches wide, and learning to row often involves a fair amount of capsizing. But the newer recreational shells are allowing more and more people to enter the sport and enjoy it right from the start. The new boats, which come in singles and doubles, are also stable in rough water that would capsize most shells, which is allowing enthusiasts to take to the water in bays, lakes, and rivers that normally aren't ideal for rowing racing shells. Recreational shells offer the same physiological benefits as racing shells.

Proper Training for Rowing

One look at the cut, sculptured physique of a rower and you'd figure these people do a lot of weight training. Not true. Studies have found that weight training, including leg presses, actually detracts from the performance of elite rowers. The weight training you do on dry land simply doesn't translate well to a boat because the fluid pattern in which power is extracted from a rower's muscles can't be replicated in the weight room. Weights leave you with chunks of specialized strength and gaps of weakness that will interrupt the graceful application of strength you need to row a boat properly.

That doesn't mean rowers don't train in the weight room, but there certainly isn't any consensus on its value. Prominent rowing programs around the world include some strength training, although volumes vary greatly. The successful U.S. men's sweep team trains 3 days per week for 30 minutes. The women's team has 2-hour sessions twice a week. The less successful U.S. men's scullers spend as much as 40 percent of their training time in the weight room.

Although coaches disagree on the value of weights, many acknowledge that weight training makes sense for novice rowers, even fit ones who arrive at the sport after years of cycling or running. Even though these athletes have strong legs, they usually have muscular weaknesses elsewhere along the rowing stroke continuum, and those weaknesses become magnified as they begin hard training in a shell or ergometer. This sometimes leads to overuse injuries. So specific weight training that develops their weak areas will help them when they get in the boat.

Older rowers—those approaching or exceeding age fifty-five—also benefit from strength training because of the natural muscle atrophy that accompanies age. Even if these mature athletes are long-time rowers, they may find that some specific weight training helps them maintain strength and muscular balance in the face of advancing age.

Stephen Seiler, a physiologist and veteran rower from Texas who is now teaching and doing research in Norway, notes that the volume of weight training rowers need is not great and should never replace the best training there is: rowing itself.

Steven Redgrave recommends that serious rowers visit the gym at least twice a week. He recommends leg presses and squats at half your body weight for lower-body strength and bench presses and bench pulls to work your rhomboids, lats, triceps, and biceps. He also recommends that rowers run at least 2 miles 3 days a week and swim 1,000 meters 3 days a week.

Although rowing is nearly injury-free, people with back problems must be especially careful to use proper technique and stop rowing if their condition is aggravated. Some doctors prescribe rowing to back patients because it strengthens abdominal muscles.

How to Train Indoors

The people who manufacture indoor rowers sometimes recommend interval workouts to break up the monotony of rowing in your dark basement in the winter. It's not bad advice, but there is evidence that steady-state rowing produces better results. Researchers in Denmark, Norway, and Italy teamed up recently to study two teams of rowers training during the summer. Both groups did the same volume of work but one team did intervals, another did straight endurance. After almost three months, the endurance team had improved their aerobic capacity an average of 8.2 percent but no significant changes were noted in the interval group. One factor in the outcome of the study might be that endurance training helps improve a rower's technique better than interval training.

Many recreational and serious rowers train on an ergometer and measure their success by their time for a 2,000-meter trial. Here are some tips on improving that erg score:

- Keep a careful log on your workouts, noting times and effort levels, how you felt, heart rate, and the time of the day in which you were working out. You may find that you get your best results in the morning or in the evening and you might want to focus your training on those periods of the day.
- Go a little further than your eventual racing distance. For four weeks, 1 day each week, stroke a 2,200-meter workout three times, with a recovery rest in between. Pace yourself on the first one and try to go as fast as you think you can maintain for the whole workout. On the next two, try going at 75 percent of your desired race pace.
- Record your meters faithfully after every piece, and any fluctuations in your stroke ratings. Estimate what kind of 500-meter splits

you have to maintain in order to achieve the same time for each 2,200-meter interval.

- Push your pace when you notice that the last piece is feeling easier and your heart rate is beginning to lower.
- After four weeks, go to three intervals of 2,000 meters at 90 percent of your desired race pace. Strive for even splits, but attempt to lower them by a couple of seconds if you're feeling especially good. On the fifth week, warm up thoroughly and then start at your desired race pace, picking up the rate slowly if you're feeling good. You could make dramatic progress.

Canoeing and Kayaking

Rowing might be the most aerobically demanding of all the boating sports, but a wide variety of flatwater and whitewater sports can challenge you physically.

Canoeing and kayaking have been Olympic sports since 1936, and today's races are contested in one- and two-person boats over 500- and 1,000-meter courses. These events are even more obscure than the

VISUALIZATION FOR KAYAKERS

Most athletes are aware of the importance of physical practice—the process of training specific muscles to work in an orderly, powerful, and efficient fashion. The more you train and practice, the smoother your actions will be and the more stamina your muscles will have.

But in such skill sports as whitewater canoeing and kayaking, successful participants need to do some mental practice as well. The mental preparation involves emotional imagery and visualization. The former strives to make you feel confident going into an event or challenging situation and the latter helps you develop a clear plan of attack before you even hit the rapids. Hundreds of studies done in recent years show that although mental practice is not as important as physical practice, a combination of the two will make you more successful than physical practice alone.

In slalom kayaking, where a race course isn't established until the day before an event, most paddlers rely on visualization to give them a better com-

rowing events, and attract such a limited number of athletes that it's possible for some competitors to have long careers. Canoeist Jon Lugbill, for instance, made the national squad at age thirteen and remained competitive into his thirties.

The training is no cakewalk. In 1990, when he was twenty-eight, Lugbill was training twice a day for up to 3.5 hours, in addition to his off-season running and weightlifting.

The whitewater side of these sports attracts more than a few daredevils. Eric Jackson, a 1992 Olympian in the whitewater kayak events and the top U.S. finisher that year at the Olympics in Barcelona, became so enamored of his sport that he sold all his worldly possessions, packed his wife and two kids in a 31-foot RV, and began a nonstop tour of the best whitewater rivers in the United States. He's gone off 45-foot waterfalls twice, and one year lost two friends and fellow competitors when they died in kayaking accidents. But Jackson keeps on kayaking. "Worry is interest on a debt you may never owe," he says with a shrug.

Recreational whitewater kayaking has grown enormously in the last several years, attracting some of the same people drawn to sky surfing

mand of the course. After a practice run or two, they fix a mental picture of the course in their heads and run through it several times on dry land. Studies show that visualizing an activity this way stimulates the areas of the brain that are used during the event itself. Sailors also use the technique.

It's not clear how much visualization and emotional imagery can improve performance. In one study of swimmers, those who used positive thinking before a swim trial improved their times by nearly 2.5 percent. In another study, older rowers improved their performance by over 1 percent when they used prepared positive thoughts before a 6-minute ergometer test trial.

When using visualization, it's important to avoid thoughts of losing or pain and to not get overly excited with visualization before a competition. Picture perfect form and a graceful effort. The simpler the better. Experiment with the technique in practice before trying it out in competition.

and other dangerous sports. The number of people killed kayaking is also growing, leading some proponents of the sport to worry that participants are trying to do too much too soon.

Canoeing and kayaking—particularly the increasingly popular sport of sea kayaking—can be much more placid, however. Although touring in a canoe or sea kayak isn't aerobically tough, it's still good exercise and a great way to work the upper body if your primary exercise is running, cycling, or walking. Jan Nesset, the editor of *Canoe and Kayak Magazine,* calls sea kayaking "hiking with your arms," and thinking of it that way makes the sport even more appealing. "You can work it as hard as you want," Nesset says. "Or you can just sit back and work at enjoying the scenery."

CHAPTER 10

SWIMMING

Mike Ryder had not swum competitively in 20 years. He'd been a talented 400- and 800-meter specialist at Arizona State, but after graduation he'd drifted away from the pool and all those 10,000-meter workouts. He'd stayed fit running and cycling, but his swimming career was essentially over.

Then one day he took his son to the pool and they noticed a flyer on the wall advertising an upcoming master's swim meet.

SWIMMING IS VIRTUALLY INJURY FREE.

Ryder's son urged him to enter. Ryder shrugged and thought, "Why not?" He joined the local master's team and got in three workouts before the meet. He won one race and took second place in two others, but he paid the price. "That night I could barely move my shoulders," he says. But the bug had bit him. "I thought, 'Hey, I'm still fast.'"

And so it was that at age forty-two Mike Ryder's career was relaunched.

Today Ryder is within a second of his fastest college time in the 100-yard freestyle and he's already equaled his college best in the 200. But he's gotten there in a very different way than twenty-five years ago. He doesn't do nearly the same mileage he once did, and he focuses much more on technique and effort level than before. After he resumed swimming, his coach monitored every stroke he took and stopped him at the wall to correct myriad flaws in Ryder's technique. "He knew if one pinkie was out of place," Ryder says. Some days all Ryder did was stroke drills, other days his pace rarely got above the leisurely level. His coaches made him stop at the wall and count his heart rate aloud, and some days that rate never got above 130 beats a minute. Other days it soared to 200. As his training progressed, his resting heart rate decreased to 46. Any morning that the heart rate was 70 or above, Ryder took the day off. In college, he never took a day off.

What's more important, when Ryder first started training, he was taking about twenty-four strokes every 25 yards. Now he's down to sixteen or seventeen strokes. He is swimming faster with fewer strokes, and in today's world of competitive and recreational swimming, there is no greater measure of a swimmer's success.

Swimming's new-found emphasis on technique is good news for anyone who is thinking about adding swimming to his or her fitness regimen. Whether you have been swimming for a long time, are returning to the sport after a long absence, or are taking it up as an alternative to the pounding of running, it's important to know that the sport of swimming has changed dramatically in recent years. With new techniques and training strategies, it's possible to improve and even become competitive again on far less mileage than swimmers used to do. Stroke drills—once considered a rest period during a workout—are a vital part of any workout and are seen by many coaches as a way to improve speed and endurance by improving efficiency. In fact, some coaches now believe that 70 percent of a top swimmer's speed is the result of refined stroke mechanics and that only 30 percent is conditioning.

The example they most often hold up is the case of Alexander Popov, the Russian sprinter who dethroned American champ Matt Biondi in the 1992 Olympic Games in Barcelona. Popov beat Biondi—considered to have one of the most efficient strokes in swimming history—by 0.2 second in the 50-meter freestyle. That's a pretty big margin for such a short race. But what was more startling about the victory is that Popov did it by taking three fewer strokes than Biondi—thirty-four strokes to Biondi's thirty-seven. "An efficiency gap of 10 percent between the world's two best sprinters was nearly inconceivable," says Terry Laughlin, author of *Total Immersion* and founder of a swimming program that emphasizes good technique over heavy training.

The notion that 70 percent of swimming speed is dictated by technique should make this sport intriguing for any serious athlete. Although aging affects our speed and endurance in many fitness activities, researchers say our ability to retrain muscles or recruit new motor units—the essence of refining swimming technique—doesn't decline with age. What's more, older athletes tend to be more patient, and patience is what's needed when you're asking your nervous system to reprogram the impulses it's sending out to get more muscles working together on a streamlined stroke.

Why Swimming Is Great Exercise

Swimming is often compared to golf or tennis because of the technical challenges it offers. But when it comes to fitness benefits, swimming has most skill sports beat by a mile. In fact, it has distinct advantages over most endurance sports, including running and cycling. Although swimming works primarily your upper body, the only sport that uses a wider range of muscles is cross-country skiing. But unlike skiing, you can swim all year 'round in a reliable, regulated environment that lets you concentrate on getting a proper workout.

With the exception of swimmer's shoulder—an aggravation of the rotator cuff caused from overuse—swimming is virtually injury free. There is no pounding. In fact, many injured athletes take to the water to maintain cardiovascular fitness while rejuvenating their muscles. Even if they are not injured, runners and cyclists can benefit by taking a day or two a week and hitting the pool. Although athletes in many sports find they can prevent overuse injuries by cross-training, swim-mers' cross-training is built in. If you are a freestyler, for instance, you can work opposite muscle groups simply by turning over and doing a

THE GREAT BODY-FAT DEBATE

Despite all the high-tech research that's been done on swimmers over the years, scientists still can't agree on one thing: Does swimming burn body fat?

Some world-class swimmers have the same body-fat composition as world-class runners. And studies show that swim training actually increased the amount of energy that can be provided from fat. One study showed it increasing 50 percent after training. Fitness author and scientist Covert Bailey says elite swimmers "tend to do aerobic, fat-burning swimming" but that women, fat people, and beginners have trouble losing fat when they exercise in water. Women and fat people won't exercise as hard because they are less sensitive to the colder temperatures of water, he says, and beginners simply aren't skilled enough to swim comfortably at aerobic levels. They find it hard to maintain momentum when breathing, so they try to increase the number of strokes between breaths. Without the oxygen they need, they wear themselves out with anaerobic exercise.

Kevin Polansky, a long-time coach in Colorado who holds a boatload of world and national age-group swimming records, says that swimming at 60 to 70 percent of your MHR will burn fat and improve your aerobic fitness. Tom Dolan, a top U.S. distance swimmer, has about 3 percent body fat, which puts him in the same lean class as any world-ranked

recovery set of backstroke. If you want to give your arm, chest, and shoulder muscles an easier day, you can do a workout with swim fins, which greatly improve leg strength and flexibility.

Swimming, particularly sprinting, can serve the same purpose as lifting weights because sprinting requires a maximal contraction of those upper-body muscle groups. Swimming isn't going to give you the cut look of a body builder, but it will beef you up in an appealing way. What's more, swimming, like walking, running, and other weight-bearing exercises, makes your bones stronger. Studies have also shown that swimming improves your lung volume more than running.

Getting Started: The Elements of (Free)Style

Good swimmers slide through the water, taking long, relaxed strokes. They never seem to tire, even when moving fast.

marathon runner. It could be that Dolan's body fat is so low because he does an abundance of long-distance, slower-paced swimming that is fueled primarily by fat metabolism and not muscle glycogen. But is Dolan unusually lean? According to Covert Bailey, male Olympic swimmers average 10 percent body fat and females 15 percent, which makes them fatter than your typical Olympic runner.

"Swimmers burn sugar, not fat," says David Costill, director of the Human Performance Lab at Ball State University and a top-notch swimmer in his own right. "Even elite swimmers probably burn carbohydrates." Costill concluded this after he tested the metabolites of

swimmers, walkers, and cyclists after they exercised at about the same level. Swimmers burned up glycogen but not fat. This finding backed up an earlier study of sixty moderately obese women who swam, cycled, or ran for 1 hour every day for six months. They all finished the regimen in roughly the same aerobic shape, but whereas the cyclists and runners lost weight, the swimmers stayed, well, buoyant. Many experts have concluded that this heavy dependence on glycogen stores explains why swimmers come out of the pool ravenous; they need to restore their energy.

Ernie Maglischo, former swimming

(Continued on next page)

Poor swimmers splash a lot and take a lot of strokes. They look like they're killing themselves.

So how do you become good? It's simple, but it's not easy.

In this section we'll take a look at how to improve your freestyle, also known as the crawl stroke. It's the most common stroke used by fitness swimmers and open-water swimmers, although many swimmers add variety to their workouts by mixing in backstroke, breaststroke, and butterfly.

The two best ways to increase swimming speed are to reduce drag and improve stroke efficiency. Long strokes use more muscles—from the back, hips, torso, and upper legs—than short strokes, which rely on smaller muscle groups in the arms and shoulders. That means that

coach at Arizona State, notes that female distance runners have less body fat than female distance swimmers, even though both groups do similar training volumes and intensities. What's more, female swimmers tend to eat less than the runners. It could be that something about swimming conserves body fat and it could be that larger women gravitate to swimming because they know they are better suited to that than running.

If you're a swimmer and you're hauling around a little extra body fat, don't despair. A little extra body fat probably isn't going to hurt you. Although many coaches contend buoyancy isn't as important as good technique and body position in the water, one study found that body fat was something of an asset, particularly for women. Women tend to gain body fat in the lower portion of the body, and this helps them float better and stay streamlined. However, men tend to gain the fat above the waist, and this can cause their upper bodies to bob higher, sinking their legs and creating drag.

According to one researcher, the ideal body fat composition for a swimmer is 10 to 20 percent for men and 15 to 25 percent for women. Maglischo estimates that anything more than 20 percent fat will create more drag than your added buoyancy can compensate for. That doesn't mean you should try to add body fat if you're skinny and you want to swim better: Too much fat increases the body's resistance in the water and inhibits its cooling mechanism. If you're a "sinker" and you want to get faster, work on your technique and you'll get faster.

if you can develop a good, long stroke, you won't tire as fast and you'll have more muscle power to draw from for speed. But also keep this in mind: The best swimmers aren't necessarily the strongest. Keiren Perkins had the weakest pull of any swimmer tested at the Olympic Games in Barcelona, but she was as sleek as a torpedo in the water and won a gold medal.

So how can you learn to swim like Keiren Perkins and Alexander Popov? Here are a few suggestions.

Keep Your Legs from Sinking

A good swimmer rides parallel to the surface, her body nicely balanced in the water. Her shoulders, hips, and legs roll with each arm stroke, and her head remains low in the water, her eyes on the bottom of the pool. One coach urges swimmers to think of their chest and shoulders boring a hole in the water and letting their legs follow. Another suggests that swimmers think of themselves swimming down as narrow a tunnel as they can fit through. It's all good advice, and it's all aimed at one important thing: reducing drag.

THE BEST WAYS TO IMPROVE SWIMMING SPEED ARE TO REDUCE DRAG AND IMPROVE STROKE EFFICIENCY.

The biggest drag for most swimmers is the hips and legs, which tend to sink. They sink because the swimmer's head is too high—it's either coming up to get a breath or it's coming up because the swimmer is looking ahead and not down. Either way, a raised head makes your hips and legs drop.

Swimming flat in the water is another way to create unnecessary drag. Next time you're at the pool, slip underwater and watch swimmers move through the water. The best are rarely flat in the water for more than a split second. Their entire bodies are rolling from side to side with each stroke, and the reason they are moving better through the water is that their bodies are more streamlined on their sides than when they are flat in the water.

Stretch It Out

The first thing you should do to reduce your dragging legs is to learn to press your chest into the water while you swim. Terry Laughlin calls it "pressing the buoy," and it's the practice of physically pushing your chest, where all your buoyancy is, into the water to better balance your body. If you use the weight of your head as a counterbalance, pushing your chest into the water brings your hips and legs up and forces the water to support them.

Emmett Hines, a masters coach in Houston, also preaches "keeping your head attached to your spine." He tells his swimmers to think of a skewer running through the crowns of their heads and through their thoraxes. If you tip your head backward, forward, or to either side, you bend the skewer and your hips drop.

Try it. Push off the wall with your arms out in front of you and start kicking lightly. Then purposefully press down into the water from your sternum to your throat, keeping your neck and head in line with your spine. When you do it right, you can feel your hips rising and your legs

POOL TOOLS: HOW THOSE GADGETS HELP YOU SWIM BETTER

The goggles you expected, but what's with those Wright brothers wings those guys have on their hands?

Those are swimming paddles, and they're just one of the many accoutrements you'll find fitness swimmers strapping on these days.

The value of most swim-training equipment is that it either increases the workload or helps make your training more specific. But most of that equipment is misused by swimmers who just want to look like they are going faster than they really are. The thing to keep in mind is this: When it comes

time for you to race, pull buoys, fins, and paddles aren't allowed. If you want to swim faster or longer, you should learn to do it under your own power.

That said, here's a quick rundown of the various training tools and an explanation of how to use them right.

- **Training paddles:** They increase your resistance in the water and therefore increase your muscular power, but unless your stroke is perfect, you can injure your shoulder. Never do more than half your workout with paddles.
- **Pull buoys:** These are tucked

popping to the surface. Now start stroking, keeping your buoy pressed into the water. It takes concentration, but it works. Back in 1937, Olympic swimmer Jack Medica called this low body position "swimming downhill," and that's a good way to think of it when you're in the pool swimming laps.

Gain Power by Rolling

Another way to reduce drag is to concentrate on rolling your body with each stroke. This might take a little longer to master than swimming downhill, but it's important that you keep trying. Your entire body, from your head to your feet, should roll in unison while maintaining a straight line in the water. The problem many swimmers run into is when they go to take a breath. That's usually when they raise their heads, and this causes their hips and legs to drop and then their nice balanced

between your legs and are helpful when you want to concentrate on your arms or when you're doing drills and don't want to be preoccupied with keeping your legs up. But they are also the preferred tool of lazy swimmers because they make swimming and turning measurably easier.

- **Fins:** These are probably the most useful of all the accoutrements because they help you stay balanced during drills and are a genuine workout. They increase ankle flexibility and leg strength but can cause swimmers to slow down their stroke rates, ruining their rhythm.

- **Kickboards:** Don't use them. They force you to keep your body flat instead of allowing it to roll. They also force you to keep your head up, which forces your legs down, another bad body position. If you want to kick, you're best off doing it on your side with your downside arm extended in front of you, turning occasionally to the other side.

rotation is thrown off kilter. Another problem is when you rotate your upper body and not your lower body, a situation that creates fishtailing and produces drag.

The best way to perfect rolling is with arm drills. Swim a length with both arms extended in front of you and stroking with just your right arm, rolling 90 degrees onto your right side as your stroking arm passes your hips and pausing on your side before beginning the recovery. Turn your head to get a breath, but don't lift your head up. Then swim a length with your left arm, rolling in the same manner. Then swim two lengths of catch-up—stroking with your right for one full stroke and then with your left, waiting for the opposite hand to return to the starting position in front of you before starting the next stroke.

ENDURANCE SWIMMING IS A GREAT WAY TO GET IN SHAPE.

One of the most common problems among swimmers occurs in the arm stroke: the dreaded "dropped elbow." The best underwater pull is one that involves not only the hand, but also the entire forearm. To achieve this, you need to flex your elbow and rotate your shoulder as you reach down and catch the water for the pull back. What many swimmers do is drop their elbows and pull through the water with just their hands. By keeping the elbow bent and at a 90-degree angle during the pull phase, you get a much bigger paddle and you recruit a wider range of muscles in the effort.

Most coaches and swimming manuals are still teaching swimmers to pull under their bodies with an S pattern. You scull out, in, and out again just before you recover your arm. But an increasing number of coaches are telling swimmers not to worry about any pattern, just pull according to your feel of the water, making sure your hand doesn't cross the imaginary line running down the middle of your body. If you are keeping your elbow flexed and rolling with each pull, you're going to tap into your greatest sources of power: your hips and torso.

One great drill for improving the size of your paddle is the fist drill. You swim a length and a quarter of the pool with your hands closed in a fist. This forces you to use your forearm for pulling. When you hit the 35-yard mark, you open your hand and finish the lap. You can really feel the extra power that comes from using a complete paddle.

Perfecting the Rhythm of Your Stroke

A big part of the balanced body equation is the rhythm and pattern of your stroke. Most people—even most good swimmers—use a windmill pattern. The right hand is entering the water just about the time the left hand is finishing its underwater pull. They stretch out the right hand, angle it downward, catch the water, and begin pulling. About halfway through that pull the left hand is at the height of its recovery, poised to hit the water and start another stroke. That's the way it's always been.

But that's changing. If you look at pictures of Popov's stroke, he always seems to have one arm extended in front of him while swimming. In fact, his stroke seems more like a relay race than a windmill; the right arm doesn't start stroking until just before the left one enters the water in front of him.

This technique, which is fairly new and difficult to master, keeps your body balanced better over its most buoyant section: the chest and lungs. Terry Laughlin teaches the technique in his Total Immersion clinics and has developed a series of drills to help swimmers learn it. Emmett Hines calls it front-quadrant swimming.

It may be some time before you can become as long in the water as Alexander Popov, but you can certainly take steps right now to lengthen your stroke. Each time you reach into your stroke, try stretching your arm out just a little longer, as if you are straining to reach for something just out of reach. Rotate your shoulder, too, and allow your body to roll. Now glide for a moment before you reach down to catch the water and start your stroke.

A variation of the catch-up drill mentioned earlier can help you keep that arm out there longer. Push off the wall with both arms extended in front of you. Start your pull with your left arm, rolling your hip away as your arm approaches it, and recover the arm fully before starting a stroke with your right arm. Breathe as you normally do, rolling your hips as the arm stroke reaches that point, and recover fully before starting the sequence over again. Do two lengths of the pool with this drill and then try adding a little snap to the exchange, starting your stroke just as your opposite arm is entering the water.

How Much Drilling Should I Do?

Because technique is 70 percent of your speed, it stands to reason that drills and technique work will take up more of your time. Emmett Hines estimates it takes 100,000 yards of drills to make a skill a habit. Terry Laughlin has seen many swimmers get 20 to 30 percent faster in just a day or two of drilling, but most swimmers should consider making a long-term commitment to stroke refinement. Why? Because you are retraining a complex system of nerve impulses and muscular responses, and if you just try to tinker with your old stroke, you'll probably fall into your old bad habits. Drills are designed to make you feel completely different in the water and trick your mind and body into thinking you are learning a brand-new skill.

You'll know your stroke is improving if you're taking fewer strokes. Swim a length of a 25-yard pool and count how many strokes you took. If you took more than twenty, you have some work to do. Some coaches even think that fifteen strokes are too many, but if you can get down in that range, you're doing very well. Many coaches have their swimmers do this drill: Swim 50 yards at an easy to moderate speed, counting your

CROSS-TRAINING WON'T HELP YOUR SWIMMING VERY MUCH

The biggest drawback to swimming is that it takes a greater commitment of time and patience than other sports. It's a difficult skill to master—even very accomplished swimmers have a tough time learning all the proper mechanics of balance and hip rotation—and it's not the type of sport that quietly accepts even short layoffs. Take a couple of days off from running and you don't lose much; take that much time off from swimming and you feel stiff and inefficient when you get back into the water. To make matters worse, there doesn't seem to be much you can do in the way of cross-training to improve your swimming when you can't get to the pool.

Still, many swimmers lift weights. Weight training will increase the amount of force a swimmer can apply to the water, and most experts agree that training 3 days a week is optimal. The exercises you select should mimic swimming motions as much as possible, including lat raises, forearm and wrist curls, bench presses, and shoul-

strokes and adding that number to your time. Now swim a set of 50s—from 5 to 10—and try to keep your score for each 50 below your original score. This drill forces you to either increase speed with the same number of strokes or decrease your strokes while maintaining speed. Either way, you're increasing your efficiency.

How Much Training Is Enough?

Some swimmers can maintain their feel for the water swimming just a couple of times a week; others feel awkward in the water if they aren't swimming at least five times weekly. Most coaches recommend that elite swimmers hit the pool no fewer than six times a week—often for two workouts a day—although there is a growing body of evidence that even elite swimmers can still improve and race successfully on a fraction of the mileage they used to do.

A good training program will be a combination of long endurance swimming (aerobic training) and short, hard swimming (anaerobic). The right mix trains every facet of your physiology, from your energy storage and energy delivery systems to your muscle structure and

der shrugs. You can even do push-ups and pull-ups, as well as squats and leg curls to improve your kick and push off the wall.

Even more popular are swim benches, which you can buy for anywhere from $300 to $800. These almost perfectly replicate the swimming motions, although you remain flat on the bench instead of rolling your hips.

A small but growing contingent of swimmers are taking up cross-country skiing as a cross-training exercise. It makes sense. Cross-country, particularly the skating technique, relies heavily on upper-body strength and uses many of the same muscle groups. If you are skeptical, try swimming sometime after taking a long cross-country ski; you'll feel like you've already done a 5,000-meter workout. The problem with skiing is that it requires a dropped elbow (tucked into your trunk and leading the way for your hand to follow through), and a dropped elbow on a swimming stroke is bad news.

neurological functions. A good swimming program makes your neuromuscular system hum like a well-tuned Ferrari, and you'll not only get faster but by most physiological benchmarks you'll hold off the effects of advancing age.

Beginners

If you want to make swimming your primary form of exercise, the American College of Sports Medicine recommends a minimum of 6,000 yards a week swum in three to five workouts at 60 percent of your maximal capacity. How hard is 60 percent? That means that if you can swim 100 yards at full speed in 1 minute and 20 seconds (you are a fairly accomplished swimmer at this rate), then you can swim those 6,000 yards in anywhere from 1:40 to 2:00 per 100 yards. At that pace and distance, your heart, lungs, and bones will enjoy great benefits and you'll probably lose some weight. Most drills will take you to that 60 percent effort level, which should be incentive for you to do them.

If you choose to make the 6,000 yards a week your goal, there are a lot of ways to make the trip there interesting. If your primary workout stroke is freestyle (it should be), mix in some other strokes from time to time to break things up. For instance, when swimming a 500, swim breaststroke or backstroke on every fourth length. When doing drills, consider getting a pair of fins; these will help you keep the speed you need to execute some of the drills and will also increase your heart rate and make it a tougher workout.

If your goal is to swim 2,000 yards three times a week, don't feel you have to swim the entire 2,000 yards continuously. You can break the 2,000 yards into smaller segments and swim each one at a faster pace, with short rests in between. For instance, try swimming four 500s or ten 200s. By swimming forty 25-yard repeats with a very short rest you can get the same cardiovascular and fat-burning benefits as you can from swimming 1,000 yards straight. These intervals allow you to play around with different speeds. Swimming long distances at the same pace day after day will train you to swim a long distance at the same pace; you'll never get faster. Breaking up your workout and adding some harder swimming will make you more fit and will make your workout more interesting.

Getting Serious

If you're looking to swimming for something more than basic fitness—if you want to start going faster or swimming longer—you need to train according to your heart rate. Keep in mind that your MHR in the pool will be 10–13 beats per minute less than when you're running.

Kevin Polansky, a world-record–setting swimmer in Colorado, became a heart rate convert after he strapped on a chest monitor during his workouts and realized why he was always feeling so tired: 80 to 90 percent of his workouts were anaerobic. He changed lanes, slowed down, and limited his hard, anaerobic work to no more than 10 percent of his workout. His resting heart rate—taken in the morning before he got out of bed—declined from 61 beats per minute to 48 beats per minute. He found he could get in shape faster and with less fatigue wearing a heart rate monitor.

You don't need to swim with a heart rate monitor—many swimmers find them to be too bulky—but you should check your pulse while resting between swims. If you do, here are some targets to hit:

- **Easy swimming** (50 to 60 percent of your MHR). This is usually your warmup and recovery rate. Keep it to 10 to 15 percent of your total yardage.
- **Weight management** (60 to 70 percent of your MHR). You can still easily talk to your lane mates at the wall, but you're burning fat and gaining vast aerobic benefits. Use this level to build a base early in the year (almost half your yardage) and decrease it as you get in better shape. Reduce it from 45 percent of your yardage to 20 percent.
- **General aerobic swimming** (70 to 80 percent of your MHR). At this rate, you're swimming some hard repeats with a rest of 10–30 seconds (longer if the interval is more than 200 yards). In doing these sets, you are training both your slow-twitch and your fast-twitch muscles, which is good for swimmers because we lose fast-twitch as we age and this will help retard that process. These sets should make up 40 to 50 percent of your total yardage.
- **High aerobic threshold** (80 to 90 percent of MHR). You're working real hard now. Lactic acid is going to become a factor. You are

swimming only a second or two slower per 100 yards than your fastest time for that distance. Keep this training to 15 percent of your weekly yardage.

- **Anaerobic or red line** (over 90 percent of MHR). You are at or near maximum speed. You'll need a much longer rest at this pace, and you'll want to limit the duration and number of these tough sets.

INTO THE DEEP: THE BEAUTY OF OPEN-WATER SWIMMING

It's a cool morning in August and about 300 swimmers are standing knee deep in the chilly water of Donner Lake. Offshore, an assortment of kayaks, canoes, paddleboards, and rowboats are gathered like a ragtag armada. Suddenly, a gun goes off and the swimmers are pouring into the water like pilgrims just off the Forty Mile Desert.

It's a scene repeated all over the country every summer. It's the open-water swimming circuit, and it takes competitors across harbors, around ocean bays, through reeds and kelp beds, across lakes, and sometimes down rivers.

Open-water events such as the Donner Lake Swim, a 2.7-mile jaunt from the east end of the lake to the west end, are to competitive pool swimming what marathon trail running is to track. It's as much an adventure as it is an endurance test, and it calls for a whole new set of strategies and tricks for success.

Open-water events are divided into three categories: the shorter swims, usually the opening legs of triathlons; medium-range swims of 1.5–3 miles; and marathon swims such as the English Channel crossing or the swim around Manhattan. Some swims, including Lynne Cox's 2.7-mile crossing of the Bering Strait in 40-degree water, don't fit nicely into any category, however.

You can usually get by with a typical 3- or 4-day-a-week pool training schedule for the first two categories, but the third category usually requires a much greater time commitment. It also requires some commitment from friends and coaches; to be successful at marathon swimming you'll probably need to do a fair amount of open-water training, which means a support boat and someone to pass you food and drink during long training swims.

Here are some precautions to take if you're planning to enter an open-water competition this summer:

- **Get used to the water.** Lake and

Different coaches recommend different levels, but they should be no more than 15 percent of your weekly yardage.

Endurance swimming—either through long, continuous swims or through interval sets—is a great way to get in shape. But if you want to compete, you'll want to add some anaerobic sprint training to your workouts. The secret to fast swimming is to improve your ability to

ocean water is usually significantly colder than pool water, so you need to get accustomed it. Unexpectedly cold water can cause your capillaries to close down (it's the body trying to keep vital organs warm and functioning), which means you won't get blood and oxygen to the muscles you want to work. This can make you short of breath and even give older swimmers a heart attack.

- **Go with the flow.** Open water has weeds, rocks, and fish, so you need to train in it so it doesn't seem threatening to you.
- **Never swim alone.**
- **Learn to swim with your head up.** Most shorter open-water competitions require that you navigate the course without the aid of a boat. Occasionally you'll have to look up to see where a marker buoy is. Good swimmers have to lift their heads only every 300 or 400 yards and they do it in a way that doesn't ruin their rhythm. Heads-up swimming definitely creates drag by forcing your legs down, but practice can minimize that effect.

- **Get used to crowds.** It's a little unsettling for some people to swim in a pack—either you're getting kicked in the face or someone is clawing up your legs. Good swimmers use the crowds to their advantage by finding other good swimmers to follow. If you can see their bubbles, you are in their slipstream and are picking up a draft from them. You can also let them do the navigating.
- **Always wear a bathing cap.** It will conserve your heat and make you more noticeable to that ski boat that might be bearing down on you. Some swimmers use Vaseline and lanolin for warmth, but some say the grease just locks the cold in. Experiment and see what works for you.

tolerate lactic acid as it accumulates in your working muscles. To do that, you swim intervals above, below, or right at your lactic threshold: the point at which lactic acid reaches critical levels in your bloodstream. In addition to improving muscle strength, sprint training will improve your muscles' buffer capacity (tolerance to lactic acid) and allow you to continue to generate energy anaerobically for a longer period of time.

Sprint training is essential for anyone who wants to swim in a meet because 70 percent of all pool events are at shorter distances that require anaerobic energy to complete successfully. But sprinting will also help out in long-distance swims, particularly in the last 100 yards of that 2-mile lake swim when your training partner has a short lead and you need a little extra to pull past him. People who train strictly at aerobic levels simply don't have that kind of explosive power.

Training volume continues to be a point of contention among coaches and researchers. Ernie Maglischo, retired Arizona State coach, recommends at least 2 hours a day but concedes that most swimmers can get by on an hour a day. Several studies have hinted that too much yardage not only has no aerobic or anaerobic benefit but actually diminishes arm power. Consequently, many coaches are trimming peak workout yardage to between 4,000 and 6,000 meters a day.

Chances are your yardage will be determined by your busy schedule, so your best bet is to try to swim as much as you can and make sure you get a good variety of training into your program. Remember: Too much endurance training hurts sprinting and too much sprinting will hurt your endurance. You need balance.

CHAPTER 11

WALKING

What got Andrew Philip going was a fun walk at his work. He and a buddy entered on a lark and they weren't out to set any records. But it bothered him to finish so far back. So the next year Philip decided to walk with more purpose. He finished second this time, his legs sore and throbbing, but he was far from through with the sport of walking. He began training harder and harder each year and honing his technique to a crisp, starched precision. After several years with a mile time stuck at 11 minutes, Philip, now in his mid-fifties, covers a mile in just 9 minutes.

DON'T FORCE A LONG STRIDE; INSTEAD, INCREASE YOUR PACE OR YOUR TURNOVER.

"I kept getting faster and stronger as I got older," the Las Vegas real estate agent says. "I saw all my friends slowing down because they weren't exercising and I just kept feeling younger."

The number of frequent fitness walkers in this country—those who participate more than 100 days per year—surpassed the number of runners in mid-1993, growing to 35 million. By 1997, the number of frequent participants had swollen to 42.8 million, with a grand total of 133.6 million Americans reporting to the Outdoor Recreation Coalition of America and the Sporting Goods Manufacturers Association that they walked for fitness sometime during the calendar year. The Outdoor Recreation Coalition determined that walking is the fastest-growing sport in the country, with a growth rate of more than 40 percent in the last 10 years. Not surprisingly, the typical fitness walker tends to be older; the average age is forty-five, as compared to the average age of frequent runners, which is twenty-six. And although the majority of walkers are women, they don't dominate the sport; 47 percent of this country's fitness walkers are men.

How do you explain the explosion? For one thing, it's something most people can do, and they can do it without specialized equipment. Consequently, walking is often the first exercise anyone ever takes up. It's one of the easiest exercises on the body, it works large muscle groups of the legs, it's something you can do with friends or by yourself, and it's something you can do just about any time anywhere. You can do it on city streets or on high mountain trails. You can do it in the snow and you can do it in the summer heat.

But walking is not without challenges. If walking is your primary exercise, it's important that you walk with conviction. Strolling is not going to give the same cardiovascular benefits of other exercise, but hard, purposeful walking will. And many of the training techniques used in other sports, such as running, cycling, and swimming, can also be used in walking. For instance, fitness walkers need to be conscious of distance and speed, and they need to consider such training methods as speed and interval work if they want to improve their overall fitness.

Getting Started

As in any exercise regimen, you should start out walking slowly and build into the session. Some walkers like to stretch thoroughly before they walk and some prefer to just stretch lightly with some static stretches of the hamstrings, quadriceps, and buttocks and save the full-scale stretching for after the walk is over and their muscles are fully warmed up. Either way, once you have worked into your walk and your joints and muscles are feeling well oiled, concentrate on gradually increasing your stride while maintaining or increasing your turnover. Both of these elements are essential to improving the quality of your workout by increasing your heart rate. And don't forget about your arms.

"So much of it starts with the arms," says M. J. Baglin, a veteran walker who rarely finishes lower than the top three in any organized walk she enters. "By turning your attention to the arms, you're actually taking a lot of pressure off the legs. The stride length and turnover just seem to come about more naturally when there is a concerted effort to work the arms."

The most efficient arm carriage is to hold them fairly close to the body, with the elbows bent at a right angle. The head is usually held high, but not stiff, with the shoulders down and relaxed. As you walk, contract the abdominal muscles to ensure a proper flow of air and to reduce the incidence of side stitches and cramps in the stomach. Think of your arms as the pendulum to the legs' stride length and turnover. Swing the arms as high as shoulder level in order to create power and to make the transition from a stroll to a determined walk. "The quicker the walk, the less stress you feel on the legs," says Baglin, who teaches race walking to beginners. "You create your own momentum."

Carolyn Scott Kortge, author of *The Spirited Walker: Fitness for Clarity, Balance and Spiritual Connection*, writes that she begins each day with a 45-minute walk with her husband. The pace for the first 15–20 minutes is conversational, but then the couple settles into silence "as we pick up the pace and get our aerobic workout," says Kortge, a fifty-six-year-old 5-kilometer and 10-kilometer race-walking medal winner at the USA Track and Field Association's National Masters Track and Field Championships. "For the next 20 minutes or so, our communication is our movement."

You can measure your effort any number of ways: with a heart rate monitor, by counting your strides (about 120 strides per minute is considered walking with conviction), or just by your own perception of effort. Walking is gentle enough that you can do it every day. But to meet the standards of the American College of Sports Medicine, you should walk 20–60 minutes three times a week at 60 to 70 percent of your MHR. If you're wondering what benefits this brings, consider this: A 30-minute walk at 20 minutes a mile burns about 120 calories. The following table describes the energy expenditure of walking at different levels of effort. Note that the faster you walk and the more difficult the course, the more calories you burn. Also keep in mind that as you progress with more and more difficult walks, your body will adapt by burning fat at increasing levels. It's the same theory of overload and progression used in any endurance sport.

	15 minutes	30 minutes	60 minutes
20-minute mile, flats	60 calories	120 calories	240 calories
20-minute mile, hills	80 calories	160 calories	320 calories
15-minute mile, flats	70 calories	140 calories	280 calories
15-minute mile, hills	105 calories	210 calories	420 calories

Getting More from Your Workout

Start with hills, and start with caution. Hills will elevate your heart rate (and reward you with a view from the top) and give you more cardiovascular and muscular gains. But at the same time, hills can be destructive. That's because downhill walking extends the knee so that it absorbs more shock from the heel strike, which increases the chance of knee pain. The advantage of downhills is that they force the quadriceps muscle on the upper front of the leg into an eccentric contraction, which means that it is stretching out as it is contracting, and any exercise physiologist will tell you that this is where real strength comes from. One bit of advice: As you are coming down, don't lock the knee and keep your leg stiff. Bend it a little as you absorb the shock. It's also a good idea to warm up before tackling the hills and to slowly build into hills by walking them only once a week for a few weeks before adding more elevation.

Walking hills should also help you improve your form. Adjust the length of your stride to the steepness of the grade; as it gets steeper, your steps should get shorter. Don't overstride because this puts too much torque on your connective tissues. Use those arms. Swing the arms with power but not out of control.

Here are some other tips to make your walk more effective:

- Stand tall, with your shoulders square and eyes leveled in front of you. Gently contract your abdominal muscles and keep your lower back flat.
- Don't force a long stride. Increasing your pace or your turnover will take care of that naturally.
- Roll your feet smoothly from heel to toe.
- Push off with the toes of your back foot to add some speed, flexing the ankle.
- Walking through sand, over rough terrain, and through shallow water will also increase the intensity of your walk.

What about weights? Weights add stress to the musculoskeletal system, which in theory should make you work harder and increase the value of the workout. One study found that walking with even light hand weights can increase your heart rate by 25 beats per minute. But the *Journal of the American Medical Association* has found that hand

> TO INCREASE THE INTENSITY OF YOUR WORKOUT, WALK THROUGH SAND, OVER ROUGH TERRAIN, OR THROUGH SHALLOW WATER.

weights can increase the chance of wrist injury and aggravate lower leg problems. Weights can also elevate your blood pressure, so if you have a problem with that you might want to reconsider using them. Otherwise, experiment. Use them once a week to start, and if it seems to have a benefit for you, keep it up and add a day every month or so. Start with light weights of a pound or two and never add more than a pound per week. No one should carry weight that is more than 10 percent of their body weight.

The best technique with weights is to swing your arms about to chest level, which will give you a more total body workout and really get your heart rate going.

Many avid walkers don't advise walking with weights. They say most walkers don't use the weights vigorously enough to gain much benefit. So they recommend saving the weights for a postwalk workout and simply concentrating on form while you're walking. If you're walking fast enough and taking on enough hills, you'll get the workout you're looking for.

This is not to say that you shouldn't lift weights at all. Upper-body weight training is as good for walkers as it is for runners, swimmers, and cyclists; weights extend your workout and increase your fat-burning metabolism.

PICKING THE RIGHT WALKING SHOE

Orthopedist Lex Simpson has seen more than his share of people who take up a walking program without giving it much thought. "You start with, 'What kind of shoes were you wearing?'" Simpson says, relating the checklist he goes over with injured walkers who come to his office. "People will stare right back at you and ask, 'Shoes? You mean I can't wear my work shoes?'

Then you ask, 'How far did you walk?' And they look back at you and say, 'Two hours. I starting feeling a little stiff and sore the last hour or so.' Most people don't realize that you can't go from maybe a 10- or 15-minute walk through the neighborhood to a 2-hour hike the first time. They need to think about what they're doing."

To start, purchase a shoe with some

When the Walk Is a Race

Race walkers, as runner and TV commentator Marty Liquori once quipped, "are the Rodney Dangerfields of track and field." That's because race-walking technique conjures up images of an exaggerated hip sway and arm movements that belong in a dance number. At the 1990 Goodwill Games in Seattle, the crowd at the University of Washington's Husky Stadium broke into laughter at the start of the men's 20-kilometer race walk. But as the smooth, arm-pumping competitors continued around the track at a 6-minute, 30-second-per-mile clip, the laughter faded into quiet awe as the men roared through the 12.4-mile race at a pace faster than most runners—even good runners—can race. By race's end, the crowd was on its feet cheering the exhausted competitors.

Race-walking technique has progressed beyond the gyrating hip movements of the early years so that the motion is very fluid and directs energy into forward rather than side-to-side motion. Done right, race walking is as smooth and elegant as running.

For that reason, race walking isn't a logical advance for all walkers because it is a sport that requires hours and hours of practice and patience before it is mastered. There are two rules to keep in mind: One foot must be in contact with the ground at all time, and your leg must be completely straight as your body passes over it. And race organizers

twist and bend. This torsional flexibility means there will be less pressure in the forefoot, where more stress is applied, than in the arch area, which is a running shoe's critical flexibility area. If you're going to use hiking shoes, they should have more support and less flex than walking shoes because of the varied and sometimes difficult terrain encountered on the trail.

Other features of a good walking shoe include the following:

- There should be sufficient wiggle room for toes.
- They should be lightweight.
- The outer sole should be stable, with enough area to distribute the weight equally.
- Use a running shoe if you can't find a special walking shoe.

are pretty strict about it; monitors are placed along the course during races and if three judges all see the same transgression, a walker can be disqualified.

Unlike fitness walking, race walking expends as many calories as running at the same speed. That's because arms play a greater role in walking than in running. The exaggerated use of the upper body means that more muscle is at work in race walkers than in runners, creating a more demanding cardiovascular workout. The other advantage of race walking is that it is much less injurious than running; the graceful stride means less pounding on the ankles, knees, hips, and feet, and the easy, erect posture explains why race walkers have fewer back problems.

DON'T FORGET TO USE YOUR ARMS.

The secret to race walking is to maintain constant velocity of the body's center of gravity. There should be little swaying or bounding. Point your feet forward and roll from heel to toe. This gliding action should be smooth and fluid, with a solid push back from the ground with the balls of feet and toes. The more firm, powerful, and efficient this push is, the more speed you will generate. As you land on the heel, the toes and forefoot should be raised about 25–30 degrees off the ground. The best race walkers maintain good flexibility in the ankles, which helps them increase the force of the push-off from the ground. In addition, they remain constantly vigilant in keeping the heel under the hips when making contact with the ground.

In the initial race walking phase, your leg will swing forward while the ankle stiffens to bring the toes up. In the next phase, called the transition phase, the knee is straightened and takes pressure off the rest of the body by absorbing weight. In the final phase, the weight is transferred to the ball of the foot.

Second, think posture and upper body. The best posture is straight and relaxed. Keep the lower back flat, with little forward or backward lean. Be careful not to bend forward at the waist. Although this can increase tempo and speed, studies have shown that such a movement creates undue strain on the lower back and actually decreases hip mobility and efficiency. Keep your head in a neutral position—that is, head up and aligned with the body. Go for the domino effect: Keep ears over shoulders and shoulders over hips. Avoid locking your head into the same side-to-side pumping action of your arms, which wastes energy. Holding your head down doesn't help either—it curtails breathing.

Keep your arms near the body. The elbows should maintain an 85-degree bend, with the hands held loose. Swing them as high as the chest but no higher. Keep the elbows pointed in to make each arm swing count. Veteran race walkers suggest starting out with an exaggerated arm swing to help you gain speed as well as to learn the motion. This action will also strengthen your upper-body muscles and will enhance their range of motion. From this exaggerated movement, gradually move to a more toned-down pumping action where the emphasis is on clean, precise movement, with the arms closer to the body.

The knee must be straight from the moment the heel makes contact with the ground until the support leg is vertical. The knee is then flexed in the recovery swing, creating more speed. Shorter strides, like short pendulums, create more turnover and more speed than longer, less efficient strides. To create even more power, plant your heel at about a 35- or 40-degree angle to the ground. As the heel edge hits the ground, tilt the foot subtly to the outside, providing a fluid movement from the heel to toe transition.

Your feet should always travel along a make-believe center line in front of you. Bring each foot down right in front of you, landing on the same line the other foot has just vacated. Serious race walkers know their hips aren't rotating fully if their feet land on either side of the imaginary center line. The hips should push forward with each stride to create a motorlike action, accelerating both the knee and the foot ahead. As the hip swings and contact with the ground is made, the heel should be slightly forward of the knee.

Training Like a Runner

Michelle Rohl knows a little bit about the staying power that race walking can give you. The two-time Olympian has raced 5 kilometers in 20:56 and 10 kilometers in 44:41. A lot of runners would like to go that fast. Rohl registered these marks during a period in which she gave birth to three children and worked full-time. During all three of her pregnancies, Rohl still trained regularly, interspersing walking with swimming workouts. In two of her three pregnancies, the low-impact nature of walking allowed her to train into her ninth month. Now that she has a family, Rohl has very little time and has to make each workout count. "Quality work is what's important, not endless miles," she says.

Like runners, race walkers mix distance or endurance training with lactate threshold training to make gains in their speed and aerobic capacity. Long workouts can extend beyond 10 miles for race walkers training for the standard 10-kilometer and 20-kilometer distances, and beyond 20 miles for those training for the 50-kilometer race. Lactate threshold for a top competitor such as Rohl emphasizes 8- to 10-mile workouts. After a 1-mile warmup, Rohl walks the next 8 miles at about an 8-minute pace, followed by a 1-mile cool-down. Speed work sessions consist of 800- to 1,200-meter repeats on the track or a measured, flat road at 10-kilometer pace.

Although accomplished race walkers can go quite fast—as fast as 6 minutes per mile—most race at 8–13 minutes a mile.

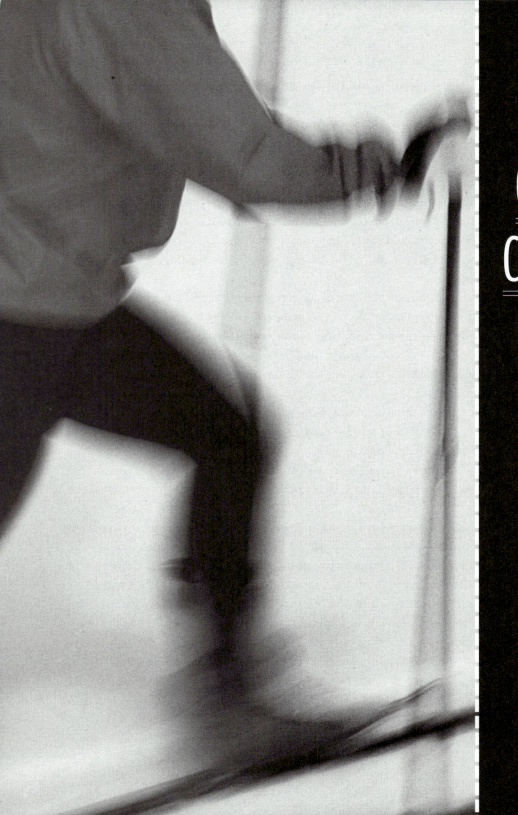

CROSS-
COUNTRY
SKIING

$\int$ kier Steven Gaskill took a class on aging and heard all about how muscle mass decreases, maximal heart rate slows down, and aerobic capacity shrinks as you get older, and it got him wondering how time would affect his cross-country skiing abilities.

So he looked up the winning times for the top ten finishers in each age group for three big races—the American Birkebeiner, the Swedish Vasolopet, and the Norwegian Birkebeiner—and found that after a slight drop in speed after the thirty to thirty-five age group, there was no significant decrease in speed among elite cross-country skiers until well into their fifties. His findings were both encouraging and discouraging.

"For a racer looking at the next several years, it is great to believe that we can maintain such high speed well into our fifties and not really see a steeper decline until our sixties," says Gaskill, author of *Fitness Cross-Country Skiing*. "Just the simple fact that eighty- and ninety-year-old skiers are racing and doing quite well, thank you, is very encouraging."

So what was it about those results that bothered him?

"The discouraging thought is that we still have to ski so fast to be competitive," he says.

It is a widely accepted axiom that cross-country skiers tend to get better with age. In fact, they improve even after they have reached the peak of their aerobic capacities. Younger skiers with the same aerobic capacities as older skiers can't seem to beat the guys who have been around for a while. Why is that? That's because the best skiers take the long view. Although many training programs build up mileage and intensity throughout the year, skiers benefit when they build up their work effort over a period of years. For instance, the Norwegians, who keep meticulous training logs, slowly increase the workload of their national-caliber skiers from 250 to 300 hours annually in their teen years to up to 1,000 hours a year in their master world-class skiers.

But even if you're not the kind of athlete who can train 3–5 hours a day, you should still see your skiing improve as the years pass. Fast and efficient skiing is the science of adjustment—of adjusting your technique, experimenting with new and better ways of waxing your skis, and breaking down the complex physics of friction and aerodynamics to find a way to get a longer glide or more power from your arms. It's said that Eskimos have more than a dozen names for snow, and most avid skiers wouldn't dispute that; the longer you ski the more you are able to discern the subtle differences in snow and how it affects your speed and technique. You may spend a week doing drills to perfect your freestyle stroke on soft, dry snow, and then it rains and freezes and the next day you find you are learning how to better edge your skis against a firm surface. The knowledge accumulates over the years, making you faster because of your ability to adjust to the conditions.

CROSS-COUNTRY SKIING IS AN IDEAL CROSS-TRAINING EXERCISE.

Studies have shown that the technique of world-class skiers is often no better than that of average citizen racers. What separates them—in addition to hours and years of training—is a veteran skier's ability to know when to switch gears, to move subtly and instinctively from one technique to another as the terrain, the wind, or the quality of the snow changes.

Cross-country skiing is a thinking person's sport, but it's also a sport that lures great athletes and can create them as well. Unlike running and cycling, cross-country skiing works the entire body, including the upper-body muscles called the latissimus dorsi, the deltoids, and the triceps. Because it is a quadripedal exercise, using all four limbs simultaneously, cross-country skiing puts the highest demands on your muscular and cardiovascular systems. It's no surprise that highest aerobic capacities ever measured in men and women came from two cross-country skiers. Studies measuring the lactate thresholds of various athletes found that sedentary people begin accumulating debilitating amounts of lactic acid when they are exercising at 50 percent of their aerobic capacity. Elite endurance athletes start feeling the sting at 80 to 90 percent of their VO_2 max. Some cross-country skiers can go as high as 95 percent of their maximum effort before lactic acid causes them to slow down—an astonishing level that reflects not only top-drawer genes but also the level of training these skiers maintain.

Although skiing can leave you with a few aches and pains, particularly if you fall, it does not pound the body the way other sports do. For that reason, cross-country skiing is an ideal cross-training exercise during the winter for many runners and cyclists. Olympic cross-country skier Carl Swenson became a top pro mountain bike

A CROSS-COUNTRY PRIMER

This chapter is not intended to teach you how to ski, but if you have never skied and want to give it a try, here are a few things you should know:

- **There are two basic styles of cross-country skiing.** The classic style is the diagonal striding technique most people associate with the sport. The freestyle technique is a newer form of skiing in which you skate over the snow. Skating is faster than diagonal striding—roughly 10 percent faster (although the gap decreases when the snow is wet or colder). One study showed that it takes 10 percent less oxygen to maintain a certain skating speed than it does to maintain the same speed while striding. That doesn't mean you can't achieve your aerobic capacity while skating—that's fairly easy to do, particularly on hills. Skating is also faster because there is reduced friction (skating skis are

waxed for total glide, whereas striding skis are waxed for glide and grip) and your body position is more aerodynamic in skating.

- **The classic style is a little easier to learn.** Not everyone agrees with that statement, but many of the movements in classic style translate to skating, so at least you're not hurting yourself starting there. Always start on flat terrain—preferably on soft, fresh snow that's been groomed—and start without any poles to help improve your balance. Former Olympian John Downing tells his students to imagine that they are children wearing socks on a newly waxed floor—push one foot forward, glide, and then bring the other foot forward and glide on it as you push off with the opposite foot. Now lengthen your glide. Now start using poles in a comfortable arm–opposite-leg

racer while he was still competing on the national ski team. Top skier John Aalberg became an All-America runner at the University of Utah while competing as a national-caliber skier. And it wasn't unusual to find three-time Tour de France winner Greg LeMond training at Royal Gorge Ski Resort while visiting his home town of Reno, Nevada. Runners and cyclists who take up the sport as a cross-training pas-

fashion, just like when you walk or run. Keep your body relaxed and start striding. That's basically it. Now you can spend the next several years increasing your glide, improving your balance, and adding a nice heel-elevating kick to the whole package.

- **Skating is easy to learn, too.** Skating is fast and glamorous. Many beginners get one look at a skating skier and immediately tell their instructors that that's the style they want to perfect that day. And if you've used in-line skates, it will be easier for you to pick it up. You start by learning the basic V-skate. While standing on a flat, groomed stretch, position your skis in a V-formation. Leave your poles by the side of the trail. Edge one ski to the inside and push off into a glide on your opposite ski. As that glide winds down, turn that glide ski inward, push off and glide on your opposite ski. Alternate back and forth, shifting your weight completely over each glide ski. When you get comfortable with this motion, add poles. In the basic skating technique, you plant both poles on the outside of your skis just as you begin pushing off your dominant leg (in this case, let's say it's the right one.) Go into the glide over your left leg as you push your arms through behind you. Kick off from that left ski and shift into a glide over your right ski, quietly recovering your arms and bringing your poles up in front of you. Plant your poles as you begin your kick and start the cycle all over again. This is called the V2 alternate. As you get better, you'll learn to pole off both legs (the V2) and offset your pole plants so you can skate up a hill (the V1). There are a few other variations you'll enjoy learning, too.

time often come to feel as though the months they spend on skis is when they do their best and hardest training.

Some History

Although ancient cave drawings suggest that humans have been scooting over the snow on skis for more than 4,000 years, most of the technological advances in skiing have occurred in the last thirty years. Race courses, which used to be just old ski trails tramped down by other skiers, are now groomed with big machines that leave behind a nicely tilled, even, grooved surface. And wooden skis have been replaced with lighter composite boards of carbon fiber and fiberglass with engineered surfaces to better absorb waxes and reduce friction. The waxes have evolved so that tins of high-tech chemical compounds can cost more than $100 each.

Techniques have also evolved. Since the mid-1970s, when a few skiers began experimenting with skis that were waxed only for glide and not with grip wax, an entirely new technique known as skating has evolved. Skating—also known as the freestyle technique because there are nearly a half-dozen variations of the basic skating stroke used by skiers—started with a few skiers leaving one ski in the tracks and kicking out with the other ski to the side (known as the marathon skate). It progressed with skiers who completely abandoned kick wax and jumped out of the striding tracks altogether to skate like hockey players over the firm snow between the parallel lanes left by grooming machines. The new techniques were embraced by America's top skiers, particularly Bill Koch, but the Scandinavian countries—where classic skiing had a long and storied history—fought it and tried to get the technique banned. Race officials put up barriers on race courses and issued bogus reports suggesting that skating was hazardous to health of women and would make men look like bulked-up body builders. None of that was true, of course.

The problem was that skiers loved skating. They carved off the tips of their old striding skis to make a better skate ski and before long the manufacturers woke up and began making specialized skating boots and skis, which have a different camber and are shorter than striding skis. Races around the world are now designated either classic or freestyle, and most serious skiers have at least one good pair of skating skis next to their striding skis in their ski bags. They also have special skating poles because that technique requires poles that are roughly 15–20 centimeters longer than striding poles.

Of course, one of the big drawbacks of skating is that, unlike the classic technique, it requires the snow be groomed. But that doesn't mean skaters aren't taking to the backcountry— many skiers have learned that spring snow encrusted by a freeze–thaw–freeze cycle is ideal for skating, and an increasing number are starting to show up on the same backcountry trails groomed for snowmobiles. Many parts of the country have extensive snowmobile trail networks that are groomed by the same type of machines used at the local cross-country resorts, and if you don't mind a little exhaust and the racket of an occasional machine, they make ideal routes for extensive skating tours. And most are free.

COMPETITIVE CROSS-COUNTRY SKIERS TEND TO GET BETTER WITH AGE.

One thing that hasn't changed much is the athletes. It's apparent from early studies that skiers—particularly Scandinavian skiers—have always been elite athletes with big hearts and the accompanying aerobic machinery. In fact, the Scandinavian countries have dominated skiing for generations, not just because they ski a lot but because they have always been fascinated with human physiology and how it affects sports performance. Scientists were out in the snow in the late 1890s using crude percussion equipment to measure the size of skiers' hearts, and their early findings showed just what you'd expect: Those with the big pumps usually won the races.

Getting Started

If you have stayed fit and are thinking cross-country skiing will help your fitness effort, you're right. But it is important not to worry too much about getting a good workout, at least not if you're a beginner. In these early stages, you should concentrate on technique. Take a lesson, or fall in with some skiers who are better than you, and practice, practice, practice. Try skiing without poles, and concentrate on committing your weight and balance to each ski. If you do this, you'll find that you are getting a great workout without even trying.

It's also important early on to stick to flat terrain. Hills might be too demanding at this stage—particularly the downhills—and the flats will give you a chance to get comfortable with the movements you'll need. Although you shouldn't go right out and buy top-of-the-line ski equipment—a package that could set you back up to $1,000—it wouldn't be a bad idea to rent performance equipment as you feel your technique come together. Good equipment won't just make you faster, it will make all the movements of cross-country skiing easier to execute. This will help you progress.

Training for Cross-Country Skiing

Most of us are happy to get out on the trails whenever we can and we don't think much about training levels and intervals and such. That's because we feel lucky just to get out and ski, and we figure the hills and our own adrenaline will provide us with all the lactic acid we need. If you're like this, getting out two or even three times a week should give you a great cardiovascular base and still leave you fresh enough to run, ride a bike, or do some other form of exercise on the other days of the week.

Some cross-country skiers are more serious, however, and they build their training programs around a simple principle: Either go really hard or go really easy. Most skiing is purposely done at easy to moderate levels—60 to 70 percent of your MHR—except when it's an interval day. On those days you go hard—at up to 90 percent of your MHR.

Most training programs call for two weekly sessions of hard intervals of 3–8 minutes in length, done at a skier's lactate threshold—the point at which lactic acid begins to seriously accumulate in his or her bloodstream (usually between 87 and 92 percent of your MHR, a level many athletes consider comfortably hard). The rest of the time they are skiing long distances at an easy pace.

The easy endurance training, as in other sports, is intended to complement the hard sessions. The easy skiing has to be easy enough that it leaves you physically and psychologically fresh for the hard training, but hard enough and long enough to produce the physiological changes your body needs to succeed. These long endurance efforts will build new mitochondrial sites in your muscles, encourage the body to push new capillaries into those muscles, and increase your muscles' fat-burning enzymes. These kinds of changes don't come with hard sessions, but these adaptations make you better equipped to handle hard sessions. One of the mistakes many skiers make is training too hard on their endurance days—they pick a course that is too hilly or they get into a pack of other skiers and start pushing the pace too much. It's easy to do that but the danger is that it will leave you too tired to do the high-quality speed work scheduled for the next day. Ultimately you wind up skiing everything at the same pace and you don't get any faster.

The hard sessions improve the body's ability to clear away lactic acid (it is gobbled up by other muscles in the body) and to buffer the lactic acid that remains. The physiological improvements you get from these hard sessions arrive quickly but they also depart quickly. That's why most skiers keep interval training in their programs most of the year, refining those sessions and increasing their intensity as they round into the racing season.

The Norwegians, who produce the best cross-country skiers in the world, limit their hard training to 15 to 20 percent of their total workloads. That leaves 80 to 85 percent for endurance training, some of which includes hidden intervals (that steep hill leading up to the lake you're trying to ski to). They try to stay away from moderately intense workouts (say in the 70 to 80 percent range) because they feel it will leave them stale for their hard workouts.

Ski coach and racer Torbjorn Karlsen recommends that hard interval skiing sessions last no more than 35 minutes, including the rest between intervals. He suggests doing four intervals of 4 minutes' duration or three at 5 minutes. He also notes that because cross-country skiing is quadripedal, the workload is greater than it is for running or cycling, even when training at the same heart rate. That means skiers use a higher percentage of their aerobic capacity because more muscles are involved in ski training—another good reason to keep your endurance training heart rate in the 60 to 70 percent range. The one exception would be if you are training only two or three times a week. If that's the case, allow yourself to bump your heart rate up 10 or 20 beats because you have all those other days to recover.

Many novice skiers—even those in very good shape from running or cycling—have a hard time staying below that 60 percent heart rate, even on the flats. Their technique isn't good enough for them to ski efficiently for any length of time. That will change as you get better. But until then, don't kill yourself to keep up with your friends. They may be in better shape or have better equipment. Just work yourself into it, concentrating on technique and walking the hills if you have to.

How Much Is Enough?

High-caliber skiers train for up to 8 hours a day, and it's not unusual for them to average more than 5 hours a day. Some of the training logs of these skiers reveal astonishing workloads—2-hour roller ski workouts followed by long trail runs, hill bounding, and maybe a weight workout. It's staggering. "Day in and day out, this schedule can really numb your sense of time and space," Olympian Luke Bodensteiner wrote in his book *Endless Winter,* a memoir about his training for the Olympics. "Workouts blend into days, days into weeks. I often find myself wondering what day it is."

The key for many of these skiers is to maintain their energy levels. Most eat high-energy snacks within 15 minutes of finishing their long workouts, and they make sure their diet is rich in complex carbohydrates and the nutrients they need to refuel and repair their bodies. Bodensteiner noted that the village housing the cross-country skiers at the 1992 Olympics consumed three times as much food per occupant as any other village. Skiers need that kind of nourishment, but they haven't always been so diligent about eating well. A study in 1985 found that many cross-country skiers were consuming only 40 percent of their calories as carbohydrates, which left them without the energy they needed to restock their glycogen stores for training. The result of that, of course, is declining performance, depression, sleeplessness, and an overwhelming sense of fatigue. So remember: Eat!

Ironically, the toughest training time for elite cross-country skiers is during the summer and fall. This is a time for roller skiing, trail running, cycling, rowing, and rock-climbing. Many skiers kayak to keep their upper bodies strong. During this time, many world-class skiers, such as Bjorn Daehlie of Norway, are training up to 25 hours a week. But when the snow flies, the racing begins and many skiers actually cut back on their training by as much as 50 percent so they can stay sharp during the December-to-April racing season.

For most of us—even high-caliber citizen racers—the winter months are usually when we bump up our training. This is when we start re-arranging our schedules and calling in favors from our spouses so we can get out on the trails for nice long, easy skis and maybe a couple of interval sessions. We don't have the luxury of long training sessions all year 'round, but skiing is so enjoyable that once you're on the trail you want to stay on it for a while. So you make adjustments.

If you have stayed in good aerobic shape the rest of the year, you can round into skiing shape pretty quickly and start racing within just a few weeks if you want to. The racing schedule for citizen racers is usually set up so that the early season races are shorter, and the longer, more demanding 30- and 50-kilometer races are later in the year.

Other training tips:

- If you're a runner or a cyclist who also likes to ski in the winter, you probably know what it's like the day after you finally get on the snow—your arms feel like they are going to fall off and your back and shoulders ache. All that can be avoided. Many skiers get a jump on upper-body conditioning by roller skiing—one effective workout is to do short double-poling intervals on a slight uphill—but even elite skiers do resistance training, either with weights or with calisthenics using their own body weight. Other skiers swear by cross-training, such as swimming, which they say uses the same muscles and gets their upper bodies in great shape for winter.

- In the summer and fall, include some hill bounding in your regular workouts. Bounding uphill is a tough workout, and it trains the body to recruit fast-twitch muscle fibers in the lower back, quads, hamstrings, and butt. Start with short (10- to 30-second) intervals with 2 minutes of rest and work up to doing 30 repetitions, pumping your arms as though you have ski poles. You can also run up hills with ski poles to develop your upper arms, and bound on flats to develop your balance and sensitivity to shifting weight from your heel to toe, just like in skiing.

- When you do hit the snow, make sure you stay on easy terrain

THE SECRETS OF GOOD ROLLER SKIING

Cross-country skiers have tried a wide variety of off-season training schemes to prepare them for the snow, but clearly, nothing works as well as roller skis.

Early roller skis were clumsy models with ratcheted wheels designed to simulate diagonal striding. Many skiers tried them, but they were difficult to master and got too many skiers into too many bad habits—real skis never had that kind of grip on snow. Although they still make roller skis with ratcheted wheels for striding, many top-level skiers won't do any striding on the roads and restrict their roller ski workouts to double-poling and skating.

The latest generation of roller skis includes models with shocks, brakes, longer-lasting wheels, and even special air-pressure tires you can take off the pavement. They'll cost you—some models are close to $300—but many skiers have found them to be the next best thing to being on snow.

Here are a few things you need to know to enjoy roller skiing:

- Ski with the flow of traffic unless your local law-enforcement agency wants you to do otherwise.

- Find an area with smooth pavement, little traffic, and modest hills that leave you some room to run out your descents. Isolated country roads are great for roller skiing, and so are bike paths and new roads into as-yet-unbuilt subdivisions.

- Wear a bike helmet. Some skiers also wear knee and wrist pads. It's

for up to six weeks. The best skiers mix skating with classic-style skiing, which is easier on the body but uses many of the same motor units as the skating technique. Many coaches feel skiers who do a lot of classic early in the season have a better technical base for the rest of the year.

- Early in the season, spend up to a half hour of each on-snow workout skiing without poles. Even if you are fairly accomplished, this will help improve your balance and appreciation of technique, and because your legs are probably in better condition from the off-season, this will give the upper body a chance to catch up without getting too sore.

always a good idea to wear bright clothing.

- Going uphill can be a great workout, but downhills can be a great way to kill yourself. Consider training with a friend. He can ride a bike up the hill while you ski and you can hold onto his bike seat while he slowly brings you downhill. Then you can switch. It makes a great interval workout.
- Always pay attention to technique. Although it closely simulates snow skiing, it's still easy to develop bad habits on the roads. Keep your feet flat on the glide, push off the glide ski evenly, and follow through with your arms. Complete motions. Do as much V2 and V2 alternate as you can to help build up your

power gears and improve your balance.

- Keep your ferrules (tips) sharp. Some skiers sharpen theirs each time out, and this is probably a good idea, particularly as the weather cools off and the asphalt gets harder. Missing a pole plant is a great way to fall or to become tentative about poling.
- Don't use your best poles. Most skiers have an old pair of aluminum poles that work great. If you have only one set of poles, go out and buy a new set of lightweight high-tech poles. Now use your old pair for roller skiing.
- Gradual uphills are a great place for strength workouts such as double-poling or skiing without poles.

- Some coaches like their skiers to take a short jog after an on-snow workout. That's usually asking a lot, but particularly if the jog is followed by extensive stretching, it will help maintain your muscular balance and full range of motion.

How to Get Faster

Although good skiers do a great deal of training, much of their speed comes from polishing their technique. Studies show that what separates great skiers from lesser ones isn't the frequency of their striding but the length of those strides. This is something you should always be thinking about, whether you are skiing as a winter cross-training workout or have made it your primary sport. Break down your movements into small parts and analyze them. How are you planting your ski? Are you following through with your arms? Try to ski with skiers who are better than you; ski behind them and try to match your movement to theirs. One difference you might notice is when they are double-poling; the better skiers tend to increase the frequency of their pole plants to gain velocity. Many skating races require skiers to double-pole the first 100–200 meters, so this skill could pay off for you.

There is no perfect body type for cross-country skiers. Whereas great runners tend to be very light and small and great rowers are tall and thick, world-class skiers range in size from 5-feet-6 to 6-feet-6. One quality of the great skiers is their upper bodies. Your arms, shoulders, and back contribute between 10 percent (classic technique) to 50 percent (skating uphill) to 100 percent (double-poling) of your velocity, so one sure way to get faster is to develop your upper body. This is particularly important as you get older and start losing some of your muscle mass to age.

If you tend to do your endurance training at too high an intensity, try to mix in some periods during that long ski when you concentrate on just using your upper body. The upper body has a lower percentage of slow-twitch muscle fiber than the lower body, and skiers have to concentrate on developing the endurance of those muscles. Studies show that Norwegian skiers aren't at their peak when their total bodies achieve their aerobic capacity but when their upper bodies have achieved their aerobic apex.

The aerobic capacity of a sedentary person's upper body is roughly 60 percent of his or her total body aerobic capacity. That means that if you are double-poling, you will reach the limit when you are consuming only 60 percent of the oxygen you consume when you reach your limit running on treadmill. With training, however, recreational skiers or citizen racers can attain 70 to 85 percent of aerobic capacity using just their arms and elite skiers can get as high as 95 percent. They didn't get there by running or even just skiing. Upper-body weight training is going to make you faster and give you more endurance for poling in cross-country skiing, and it's particularly important for older athletes.

Don't expect to slow down much as the race lengths increase. You'll find that you won't have to. Ski racers can maintain their speed over longer distances than, say, runners can. The top runners are 19 percent slower in a marathon than they are in a 5-kilometer race, whereas skiers moving from a 10-kilometer classic race to a 50-kilometer race lose only about 5 to 7 percent of their speed. Why is that? It could be that the longer ski courses are not as hilly (per kilometer) as the shorter ones, but it may also be that skiers, because they use the entire body, have more total glycogen available to create energy.

And keep in mind that cross-country skiing technique—at least the freestyle technique—is still developing. For instance, for years instructors have been telling accomplished skaters to align their noses, knees, and toes as they shift weight from one ski to the next. They've also been telling them to ski a flat ski, meaning that they should try to keep their glide skis flat as they move their bodies over it. But now new studies, based on the video analysis of Olympic cross-country skiers, show that the best skiers don't pay much attention to the nose–knee–toe alignment and don't spend much more than a split second on a flat ski. They concentrate instead on smoothly moving from one ski to the next, emphasize propelling themselves down the trail rather than on their lateral movements, and swing their arms to shift their weight from ski to ski.

Knowing your gear and waxes will also help. As in rowing and cycling, your equipment goes a long way to determine how fast you'll go and how quickly your technique will improve. Good equipment—skis that are the right stiffness and length for your weight—improves your balance and the length of your glide, two keys to successful skiing.

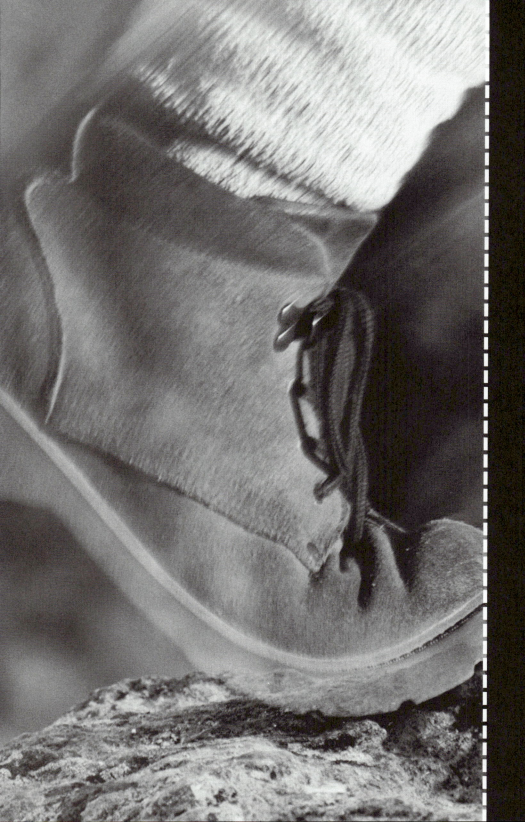

HIKING

During his pursuit of the world's first sub–4-minute mile in 1954, Sir Roger Bannister often retreated to the mountainous country of North Wales for long hikes that took his mind off the intense training he was doing. What Bannister found was that hiking helped build strength and endurance that paid off when he ran that historic mile race in 3:59.4. Later in life, as a cardiologist, Bannister recommended hikes to his patients as a way to build confidence and fitness.

STRENGTH TRAINING CAN HELP AVOID SORENESS AND INJURIES.

Just as runners often turn to trails to add variety to their workouts, many walkers find that hiking heightens their sense of satisfaction in their sport. When you are out walking on a city street or sidewalk, the world passes by like a movie. When you are out on a remote hiking trail, you become the star of the movie.

That is because hiking has an element of exploration to it, whether it is the vistas that spread out unexpectedly when you reach a high-elevation meadow or that glimpse you catch of wildlife scurrying off the trail in front of you. "You can't buy the scenery you see," says fifty-four-year-old Tom Wright, who hikes on the trails of the Sierra Nevada gold country in California. "In just a few miles, you can venture places few other people have ever been. It makes you feel privileged. And it makes you feel like you've earned the privilege."

In this regard, hiking is better than almost any other form of exercise. It simply takes you places few people go, and in this day and age, when stress, anxiety, and depression cause employees to lose an average of 16 days a year from their jobs, that quality is indeed priceless.

In addition to the emotional satisfaction, there is the physical satisfaction. Hiking offers all the physiological rewards of walking and more. For one thing, most hikers are carrying some extra gear, whether it's a fanny pack, water bottle, or fully loaded backpack, and that can add dramatically to the cardiovascular workload of the activity. What's more, because hiking trails are often uneven and have irregular surfaces, your body is continually having to recruit new motor units in order to maintain balance and momentum.

It's no surprise, then, that so many people are turning to hiking as their primary form of exercise. In 1997, there were 47.7 million hikers in the United States, and an additional 15.2 million backpackers. More than 20 million of these folks were over the age of forty, including Emma Gatewood, a sixty-seven-year-old Ohio grandmother who hiked the 2,160-mile Appalachian Trail in sneakers while carrying her gear in a duffel bag.

Getting Started

The mistake many hikers make is not adequately preparing for the demands of the sport. "They limp in on a Monday morning saying they're sure they tore a calf or quad muscle," says physical therapist Randy Jacobe. "Then they happen to mention that they hiked to the top of a 10,000-foot mountain over the weekend. When you ask them what special preparations they made for what is the equivalent of climbing and descending hundreds and hundreds of flights of stairs in a single day, they usually say, 'None.'"

Until you can get out on the trail, you have a variety of methods for getting in shape for those tough hikes and backpacking trips. Walking, of course, is the best exercise to start with. Gradually build up from 2–3 miles an hour to where you are walking 2 miles in 30 minutes or less. From there, either increase the distance or start adding a route that has hills. You can add both distance and difficulty, but you run the risk of doing too much too soon and getting injured. Build slowly and always give yourself time to warm up properly. And whether you are a beginner or an expert walker, remember to stretch after your workout, while your muscles are still warm.

More fit hikers add even more levels of difficulty to their preparation. It's not unusual these days to see people using stair machines wearing full backpacks. Some hikers strap on a full pack and then climb the stairs at their local football stadium, a workout that gets them used to both the uphill portions of their upcoming hike and the downhill parts. Ironically, it is the downhill sections—the stretches of trail you'd think were the easiest—that leave more beginner hikers feeling sore in the days immediately after a hike. That's because downhill walking requires an eccentric contraction of the quadriceps muscle; that is, it is lengthening at the same time it is contracting. It's great exercise, but it can leave you very sore and the only way to avoid it is to practice the activity that causes it.

Hikers should follow the same progression and overload principles used by any fit person or athlete. They should also follow the principle of specificity. What all this means, of course, is that you don't wait until you are at the trailhead to strap on a backpack for the first time that year. If you are planning a major hike or backpacking trip for the spring, for instance, you need to gauge how hard this will be and work back from your target date and develop a program that will get you ready. And that program should be designed to challenge your body, with increasing levels of stress and the requisite periods of recovery, in the same way it will be challenged out on the trail.

Say you are planning a 5-day trip into Desolation Wilderness. You might be hiking 5–8 miles a day with a 50-pound pack. In the weeks and months before that trip, you will need to make sure not only that you are comfortable hiking those distances (with those kinds of hills) but that you are also ready to carry the weight. Some suggestions:

- Get the pack out, add some weight to it, and start walking, even if it's around the neighborhood for a few miles. As the weeks pass, add more and more weight until you are comfortable with carrying 10 pounds more than you expect to have in your pack during your expedition.

- If the weather's bad, hike on a treadmill or stair machine, set at the kind of intensity you hope to hike at. If you aren't in very good shape, start at a comfortable pace at which you can still carry on a conversation. But as time goes on, add some intervals that leave you feeling somewhat winded. When those intervals become comfortable, increase the speed or incline of your treadmill or the resistance of your stair machine.

- Get out on real ground as soon as you can. Indoor machines are great, but there is nothing like getting out into the woods to add some variety and inspiration to your workout. Even if it's only once a week, that hike in the woods will make all your indoor workouts more bearable.

- Some hikers like to do their preparation workouts with leg weights on. These seem to work best when you're outdoors and hiking up hills because they don't add a great deal of stress to your joints and can make your legs feel light when you finally get out on the trails.

There are some physiological benefits from hiking with a backpack. For one thing, you use a wider range of muscle groups, so you are burning up more calories. For instance, a 140-pound person carrying a 5-pound pack burns 310 calories an hour and a 185-person carrying a 20-pound pack burns 500 calories an hour, on average.

Although we take our walking technique for granted—after all, we've been doing it since we were toddlers—converting your regular walking stride into a hiking stride can cause you some trouble. Be wary of overstriding, particularly if you are wearing a backpack or fanny pack, because that action can stress your shins and leave you sore. Find a natural gait, and if you want to pick up your speed as you get in better shape, increase the pace, not the stride length. Stretching will naturally lengthen your stride for you. Also, think about your breathing: Rapid, shallow breaths may feel natural as you're making your way up that 10 percent grade, but longer **and deeper** breaths will help you deliver more oxygen to your hungry muscles.

You may be in great shape, but it's always important when starting out on a hike to warm up properly. This is not a forced march, and you will enjoy the hike more if you work slowly into your pace. And at the end of the hike, before you pile into the car, take the time to do some stretching. If you wore a backpack, stretch your upper body and walk around for a while without your load.

When getting ready for a specific hiking or backpacking trip, it's important to be realistic. If you have a busy schedule that allows you to exercise for only 45 minutes three or four times a week, don't plan on climbing Denali. At the same time, if you've got your heart set on doing the Pacific Crest Trail, allow yourself adequate time to prepare. Start slowly and build up slowly over a long period of time. Give your body time to rest and repair itself.

Strength Training for Backpackers and Hikers

You can avoid the sore back and shoulder muscles that usually accompany the first hike or backpacking trip of the season by doing some weightlifting before you get out on the trail. In addition to preventing soreness down the road, weightlifting will hold off the loss of muscle mass that accompanies aging. Although you can follow a general weight program prescribed by a trainer or set out in a class at the YMCA, here are some exercises using a 5- to 15-pound dumbbell that all hikers should include in their regimens:

- **Arm curls:** Hold the dumbbell at your side with your palm facing forward. Curl the weight up to your shoulder slowly and then curl it back down. Do that to failure; if you can easily go past ten repetitions, add weight until ten is the most you can do. Switch arms and then repeat with the palm facing backward.
- **Bending lateral arm lift:** Bend at the waist until your upper body is parallel to the floor and the dumbbell is hanging straight down. Keep

HIKING INJURIES

It's May and you've just completed your first big hike of the year. You feel great—you reached that 10,000-foot peak in a single day—but you're worried because the fronts of your legs, from your knees to your ankles, are throbbing and sore.

Don't despair. That pain you're experiencing is probably just good old-fashioned shin splints.

A wide variety of lower-leg ailments fall into the category of shin splints. The pain runners often experience, for instance, is typically an inflamed tendon, and sometimes that injury takes a long time to heal. The shin splints walkers (and to a certain extent cross-country skiers and snowshoers) experience is usually a sore muscle, the result of the tibialis anterior muscle not being strong enough to handle the stress you're heaping on it.

Here are some tips for getting over your pain faster or preventing it in the first place:

- If the pain is not severe, you can continue to exercise. The pain will subside once the muscle gets heated up and if it returns afterward, try icing the area and taking ibuprofen.
- Sit on a table or chair and loop a weight around your foot. Without bending at the knee, move your foot up and down at the ankle to strengthen the muscles and the tendons.
- Stretch your calf muscles. Tight calves can stress the anterior leg muscles.

the elbow locked and slowly lift the arm to the side. Do 5 to 10 reps.

- **Arm lift:** Hold the dumbbell at your side, palm facing backward. Lift forward, elbow locked, until arm is parallel to the floor. Slowly return to side and repeat.
- **Lateral arm lift:** Hold dumbbell at your side, with your palm facing the body. Lift the arm out from the side, with the elbow locked, making sure to lift it not much higher than parallel to the ground. Gently lower the weight back to the starting position. Repeat 5 to 10 times.

Finding the Right Pace for Your Hike

Finding the right pace is difficult for many hikers. Some hike too fast, get winded, and have to stop. Depending on how fast you were

- Get the right shoes. Shin splints are often caused by poor-fitting or worn-out shoes. Be careful not to hike in running shoes, whose heels are often built too high for hiking. If trouble persists, see a podiatrist about orthotics, a shoe insert to control poor foot motion.
- Walk on your heels periodically through the day. Race walkers actually do intervals—usually not more than 30 seconds long— walking on their heels.
- Work your toes. Spell the alphabet with your toes while you're sitting in a meeting or reading at night.

  Some hikers who overdo it develop a condition known as plantar fasciitis, which occurs when the plantar fascia— the tissue that connects the heel to the base of the toes—becomes inflamed or torn. It's a dull and occasional pain that, if left untreated, can become a sharp and constant pain. Plantar fasciitis is not a condition to take lightly. It can take up to a year to heal and often interferes with whatever exercise program you're on. If you have this kind of pain, see a podiatrist. He or she will probably prescribe some stretching exercises and ask you to wear a splint or boot to immobilize the area. Some people get cortisone shots to relieve the pain until stretching and other forms of physical therapy can help. Few patients—less than 2 percent—need surgery, and many hikers prone to plantar fasciitis find relief in $10 heel pads you can buy at the pharmacy. One study found that those heel pads work better than $400, custom-made shoe inserts.

hiking, sudden stops from a crisp pace could contribute to soreness the next day. So it's important to find your rhythm.

Whether you are hiking or backpacking, start out slowly and work into a steady pace. You're not in a race, but if the hike is to have any fitness benefit, you should feel slightly winded, though able to carry on an easy conversation. If you find you are working harder than that, don't suddenly stop and rest, but slow down to the point where your heart isn't racing quite as fast. If you find yourself speeding up and becoming breathless again, slow down again. Eventually you'll develop a sense of pace that works for you, and as the season progresses, you'll be able to pick up that pace.

You can also borrow a trick from runners and pay attention to the pace of your breathing. If you are inhaling and exhaling on every other step, you are probably hiking too hard. But if you are inhaling slowly and exhaling on every fourth footfall or so, you are probably working at a level that is slowly burning sugar and fat—a pace that will give you the energy you need to keep going for hours. If you are exhaling every third footfall, you might still be burning fat but you're probably burning primarily sugar and will bonk within a couple of hours.

Concentrating on your breathing rhythms might also help your efficiency; keep your stride steady and your stride length consistent, even on a steep or rutted trail. When you reach a tough section of trail, focusing your attention internally—on your breathing pattern—is a good way to keep moving without debilitating fatigue. Elite athletes use a method called belly breathing in which they call on both the diaphragm and abdominal muscles for moving air in and out of their bodies, a method that seems to deliver a greater supply of oxygen to working muscles.

Get Good Gear

Good gear is important in any sport, and hiking is no different. You may not need those heavy-soled boots they sell mountaineers, but you will need a shoe that gives you support, durability, and traction. Running shoes may not be sturdy enough, but lightweight trail shoes are almost as comfortable and don't take as much energy to haul up the mountain as those heavy leather boots we wore years ago.

When it comes to boots, pick a pair that are comfortable right out of the box. They shouldn't have to be broken in. Blisters are probably the main cause of prematurely terminated hiking and backpacking trips.

Look for shoes with solid ankle support because the trail will turn into a jumble of twists and turns at some point. The most durable and versatile hiking shoes usually have a firm, waterproof full-grain leather upper. Look for boots with very few seams; one-piece uppers usually provide the best water resistance. A nice feature of many hiking boots is what is called a gusset, or a thin strip of leather sewn to the upper and the tongue. The gusset serves as a shield against rocks and water, the primary culprits for blisters.

Shop around and don't cut corners when it comes to hiking boots and socks. All-cotton socks can get wet, bunch up, and leave your feet blistered. Also, make sure your socks fit snugly. You can also rub Vaseline in places that are susceptible to blisters, such as heels and between your toes. Keep your toenails trimmed.

Pick the rest of your clothing with equal care; look for materials that can wick sweat away from your skin, and always dress in layers. Many hikers break a heavy sweat on the way up and reach the top soaking wet, only to find it 20 degrees cooler. Shed the clothes as you go up and add them as needed as the temperature or your effort level drops. Always expect the worst.

Snowshoeing

Snowshoes have been around for 6,000 years, but only in recent years have they become a popular winter recreation and training activity. That's because a new generation of lightweight, easy-to-use snowshoes has become available. Now, backcountry trails once traversed in winter only by a few talented backcountry skiers are now accessible to snowshoers of all abilities.

Unlike cross-country skis, snowshoes have a very short and gradual learning curve. If you can walk, you can snowshoe. What's more, you don't need a packed or groomed trail, you don't have to worry about wax, and, if you're using ski poles, you can make your trek as physically demanding—and rewarding—as a cross-country ski.

Modern-day snowshoes come in a variety of forms:

- Backcountry shoes, which are wide and long (usually 8 inches by 30 inches) and can help you slog through just about anything. They also weigh more—up to 3 pounds—but they are essential if you want to make progress through the really deep stuff.
- Recreational snowshoes, which are shorter, lighter, and cheaper and are good for casual hiking.
- Cross-trainers, which, like the shoes, aren't great at either end of the spectrum they try to span. They are just a little too long (26 inches) for high-performance running and don't have the surface area you need for expeditioning.
- Racing models are the narrowest and shortest of all the shoes (roughly 8 inches by 25 inches) and are best on firm-packed or crusty snow where what you really need isn't so much a platform as stability.

Of course, a big part of your enjoyment on snowshoes will be dictated by the shoes you wear. The secret here is to get in the most comfortable shoes you own and make sure you can keep your feet dry. If you're wearing a hiking boot in your snowshoe, it's a good idea to wear gaiters to keep snow from falling down inside and melting around your socks. If you're wearing lightweight running shoes, consider getting a pair of neoprene booties to keep your feet dry.

After that, it's as easy as walking. Once you're out on the trail you'll find that snow conditions dictate the type of workout you do. If the snow is soft and you're on racing shoes, it's probably going to become too much of a struggle to run. You can still get a good workout just by slogging through (poles will help boost your heart rate), particularly if you chose a hilly route. And striding downhill through deep snow is a blast in snowshoes.

On firm, stable snow, you'll have an easier time running or walking hard with poles. Many snowshoers carry poles with them, running segments without poles and then walking tougher segments using the poles. This is a good way to extend the length of your workout because using your arms gives you access to a greater amount of glycogen. You're also building endurance over a greater number of muscle groups.

Although you can strike off just about anywhere you want to go in the woods in the winter, it's still a good idea to stay on established trails you are familiar with. For one thing, you're less likely to get lost if the trail is marked; for another thing, it's easier to damage vegetation that is off the beaten path. It's not hard to set a manzanita bush back a couple of years by crushing it under a snowshoe when a soft drift gives way. And don't worry about being bored with the same old trail you run or mountain bike on; one of the beautiful things about winter is that it transforms the landscape and opens up vistas you didn't notice last summer.

WARM UP PROPERLY.

Even if you are using snowshoeing as a fitness activity, it pays to think like an expeditioner. Make sure you're carrying matches, extra dry clothes, plenty of water, and some high-carbohydrate snacks. If you're snowshoeing alone, make sure someone back home knows where you're headed.

Variations of Hiking

The increasing popularity of hiking and backpacking has spawned a number of offbeat variations of the sport. Foremost among these are fast packing, bushwhacking, and rugged walking.

Fast packing is the sport of conquering long hikes—such as the 21.4-mile round trip to the summit of 14,994-foot Mount Whitney— far faster than most hikers. Fast packers travel light, carry potent, high-energy food, measure out their water, and cover routes such as Mount Whitney in 1 day rather than the 2- or 3-day ascents most hikers attempt. Fast packers, alternating between running and power walking, can do the double-crossing of the Grand Canyon—a hike that requires 12,000 feet of climbing and 12,000 feet of descending—in less than 10 hours.

Rugged walking is an equally exhausting activity in which hikers treat the natural environment as what Patricia Kirk, author of the book *The Rugged Walker*, calls "the ultimate exercise studio." Rugged walkers basically prowl the terrain looking for something to leap, lift, or lunge after. They sprint up grassy slopes, do lifting exercises with boulders they find beside the trail, or do bounding exercises to get across a swollen stream. "Use nature's terrain as training ground and its beauty as inspiration for a variety and cross training in order to keep exercise fun, challenging and well-rounded," Kirk says.

Bushwhacking combines the strenuous labor of fast packing with rugged walking's spontaneity. The idea is to leave the established trail and strike off on your own into areas not populated by hikers. You can see more wildlife this way and your hike becomes a little more adventurous. Not only do you need to be in excellent condition, but you need to know how to use a compass, topographic map, and even a global positioning system. Because bushwhacking can leave you lost or staring at the level gaze of a grizzly, you should always travel with a partner, alert friends or family where you are going, and carry some emergency equipment, including first aid, clothing, matches, a water filter, and extra food.

ALTITUDE SICKNESS

There is a tradeoff for hiking up to high places: You get great views but you have to look at them through thin air.

High-altitude sports physiology studies show that as we go up in altitude, we impair our ability to exercise. The reason: decreased oxygen. A study from the Northern Arizona University Altitude Sports Training Complex indicates that it takes about two weeks to fully acclimatize to elevations of 6,000–6,500 feet from sea level. No wonder that acute mountain sickness (AMS) can be a threat to the day hiker who tries to reach a 10,000-foot peak in a day.

The occurrence and severity of AMS are related to the altitude, speed of ascent, physical exertion, and time spent at altitude. The symptoms of AMS include headache, shortness of breath, nausea, weakness, and flulike malaise. The best advice is to start slowly and to avoid overexertion. If possible, spend a night or two at the high-elevation trailhead before attempting your hike up into the thinner air. Even 24–48 hours of sleeping and eating at 6,000 feet will help you when you get to 10,000 feet. But above all else, avoid alcohol, sleeping pills, and narcotics; if you're going to drink a lot, make sure it's water. Dehydration occurs more quickly at higher elevations.

If you're stricken with AMS, drink plenty and return to lower elevations. Emergency room physicians in Summit County, Colorado (elevation 9,000 to 12,000 feet) report that a quick return

Rogaining is an obscure sport but it is extremely challenging from both a mental and a physical standpoint. Rogaining involves teams of two to five people who use cross-country navigation in an effort to visit as many checkpoints as possible in a 24-hour period. Although elite orienteers, such as those on the Swiss or Norwegian national teams, are often top-flight athletes who can think clearly when their hearts are pounding at near-maximum levels after a run through a thick forest, rogaining attracts people from all ages and fitness levels. Whereas some teams are very athletic and cover as much as 100 kilometers (62 miles) in a 24-hour period, some teams may walk only 10 kilometers. The pleasure comes not only from the physical exertion but from the intellectual satisfaction of finding your way accurately through the wilderness.

to Denver (elevation 5,280 feet) will almost always alleviate minor AMS symptoms within a day.

Older climbers appear to be less vulnerable to AMS. A recent study in *Annals of Internal Medicine* suggests that people over sixty are only half as likely to develop AMS as people between twenty and thirty-nine. "We don't yet know why that is," says eighty-one-year-old Charles Houston, a well-known climber who helped write the study.

A more serious condition is called high-altitude pulmonary edema (HAPE), which takes up to 3 days to occur and is characterized by a cough with congestion, difficulty breathing, confusion, and shortness of breath. HAPE can sometimes be fatal. Sufferers should be moved to lower elevations, hydrated, and rested for a few days. Physicians tell the difference between AMS and HAPE by measuring blood oxygen levels. At sea level, oxygen saturation is 98 to 100 percent. Those with AMS have only 80 to 90 percent. Levels below 80 percent bring on the confusion and lack of focus associated with HAPE.

Researchers at the University of Innsbruck in Austria have found that 20 to 50 percent of skiers and mountaineers get headaches when they reach elevations above 9,000 feet. But they found that taking aspirin before and during the trip can help prevent these headaches.

Bouldering

Many hikers find themselves in some pretty steep country that requires them to use their arms as much as their legs. This is where hiking changes from an aerobic exercise into a strength exercise (although depending on the pitch of the climb it can be both aerobic and strength-building) and these areas are a great way to build your overall fitness and your sense of satisfaction. Actually, climbing with arms and legs without support ropes has recently become a sport in its own right. It's called bouldering and it's the activity that often converts hikers into rock climbers.

Technically speaking, bouldering is the art of practicing climbing skills without a belay. It's usually done at the base of cliffs or in areas of large boulders where climbers can practice climbing techniques just a few feet off the ground where they won't be hurt (badly) if they fall. Beginner rock climbers use these areas to practice and build up the courage to lead on a rock face, but even veteran climbers use bouldering as a way to stay in shape when there aren't any climbers around to pair up with.

Hikers should be cautious if they encounter a cliff with bouldering possibilities. It pays to go out the first couple of times with someone who knows what he or she is doing and can teach you a few holds and act as a spotter on the ground as you climb. Many beginner climbers bring mats to bouldering areas so they can be assured of having a soft landing if the rock crumbles in their grip. It might also be a good idea to practice climbing in a safe, regulated climbing gym before attempting any bouldering expeditions.

Many hikers won't be interested in bouldering, but others might find it to be the perfect transition from their love of hiking in the mountains to their dream of conquering even tougher routes requiring technical rock climbing. And even others may be drawn to bouldering because it improves your sense of balance and coordination while improving your overall strength.

SELECTED REFERENCES

Bailey, Covert. *Smart Exercise: Burning Fat, Getting Fit*. Boston: Houghton Mifflin, 1994.

Ban Breathnach, Sarah. *Simple Abundance*. New York: Warner, 1995.

Bergh, Ulf. *Physiology of Cross-Country Ski Racing*. Translated from Swedish by Michael Brady and Marianne Hadler. Champaign, Ill.: Human Kinetics, 1982.

Carlson, Richard. *Celebrate Your Child*. San Rafael, Calif.: New Woren Library, 1992.

Carlson, Richard. *Don't Sweat the Small Stuff*. New York: Hyperion, 1997.

Carlson, Richard and Joseph Bailey. *Slowing Down to the Speed of Life*. New York: Harper Collins, 1997.

Cooper, Kenneth. *The Aerobics Program for Total Well-Being*. New York: Bantam Doubleday Dell, 1985.

Costill, David L., Ernest W. Maglischo, and Allen B. Richardson. *Swimming*. Boston: Blackwell Scientific, 1992.

Dervin, Dan. "Sports, Athletes and Games in a Psychoanalytic Perspective" in *Mind–Body Maturity*. Edited by Louis Diamant. New York: Hemisphere, 1991.

Diamant, Louis, ed. *Mind–Body Maturity: Psychological Approaches to Sports, Exercise, and Fitness*. New York: Hemisphere, 1991.

Healy, Jane M. *Endangered Minds: Why Our Children Don't Think and What We Can Do About It*. New York: Simon & Shuster, 1990.

Jerome, John. *Staying Supple: The Bountiful Pleasures of Stretching*. New York: Bantam Books, 1987.

Jerome, John. *Staying With It: On Becoming an Athlete*. New York: Viking Press, 1984.

Kiesling, Stephen. *The Shell Game: Reflections on Rowing and the Pursuit of Excellence*. New York: Morrow, 1982.

Kirk, Patricia. *The Rugged Walker*. Champaign, Ill.: Human Kinetics, 1997.

Kortge, Carolyn Scott. *The Spirited Walker: Fitness for Clarity, Balance and Spiritual Connection*. San Francisco: Harper, 1998.

Laughlin, Terry. *Total Immersion*. New York: Simon & Shuster, 1996.

Maglischo, Ernest W. *Swimming Even Faster*. Mountain View, Calif.: Mayfield, 1993.

Noakes, Timothy D. *The Lore of Running*. Champaign, Ill.: Human Kinetics, 1996.

Ostrow, Andrew C. *Physical Activity and the Older Adult: Psychological Perspectives*. Princeton, NJ: Princeton Book Co., 1984.

Sobel, David and Robert Ornstein. *Healthy Pleasures*. Reading, Mass.: Addison-Wesley, 1989.

Walford, Roy L. *The Anti-Aging Plan: Strategies and Recipes for Extending Your Healthy Years*. New York: Four Walls Eight Windows, 1994.

Waterhouse, Debra. *Outsmarting the Midlife Fat Cell*. New York: Hyperion, 1998.

Wescott, Wayne. *Strength Training Past 50*. Champaign, Ill.: Human Kinetics, 1997.

Zelinski, Ernie. *The Joy of Not Working*. Berkeley, Calif.: Ten Speed Press, 1997.

Web Sites

There are too many great sports and health sites on the Internet to list here, and half the fun is finding them yourself. But here's a few I came across while researching this book. I found myself returning to them again and again to verify information and stay on top of new research developments.

wwilkins.com/MSSE/. *Medicine & Science in Sports & Exercise* (official journal of the American College of Sports Medicine). Really technical, but has a lot of great research material you can read through and search.

Phys.com. Good site for general questions about fitness and diet, geared toward women but helpful to men, too. Includes information from *Vogue, Glamour, Mademoiselle, Self, Allure*, and *Women's Sports and Fitness*.

kicksports.com. Good overall running site, with information on running clubs, injuries, training, calendars, virtual races, eating, gear, and cross-training.

krs.hia.no/~stephens/index. The Masters Athlete Physiology and Performance page gives you detailed, sometimes technical and sometimes folksy information on rowing, cross-country skiing, running, cycling, and other endurance sports. Good site for the elite athlete who wants to know the why as well as the how. Written by an American exercise physiologist who is doing research and teaching in Norway. Ideal for the older athlete.

Sportquest.com. Detailed, searchable resource center that helps make sense of the wide variety of sites on the Web dedicated to sports, fitness, nutrition, and health. A good starting point.

Sporstsci.org. Sportscience, an interdisciplinary site for research into human performance. The page is hosted by the Royal Society of New Zealand but has a lot of practical information based on solid scientific research. Very easy to understand. The archive is searchable.

Peakrun.com. Peak Running Performance has a wealth of running articles, quizzes, and training tips. Information runs the gamut from raising your lactate threshold to improving your race performance with age.

Runnersworld.com. The popular magazine's Web site has daily news, the tip of the day, and full-length articles culled from the magazine. Also has the obligatory training tips for all types of races, from 5-kilometer runs to marathons. There is even a good beginner's program.

Mindspring.com. Has links to The Webwalker, a good jumping-off point for the experienced or beginning race walker. Has age-graded tables and articles on hiking. Great spot to get in touch with clubs and organizations if you're traveling and need workout partners.

Physsportsmed.com. The Physician and Sportsmedicine Online is a good source for primary care sports medicine and clinical and personal health articles. This is also a good link to other sports medicine sites.

Mayohealth.org. The Web site for the Mayo Clinic is a tremendous resource for the latest on general health issues. Is caffeine bad for you? How can you test yourself for testicular cancer? It's an extensive, easily maneuvered site for general health information. Also check out **healthanswers.com.**

Getting Measured

A number of sites offer you instantaneous calculations of various physiological standards. One of the more interesting is the VO$_2$ max site (**sirius.on.ca/running/vo2.shtmlanchorcal/**). Click to **lactest.com** to find out how you can get your lactate threshold tested by mail.

INDEX

ABOUT THE AUTHOR

Jim Sloan lives in Truckee, California, with his wife, Karen, and their two daughters, Emma and Lily. He is an active cross-country skier, trail runner, cyclist, and open-water swimmer, and has written extensively about health, fitness, and environmental issues for various newspapers and magazines on the West Coast. His first book, *Nevada: True Tales from the Neon Wilderness*, was published in 1993 by the University of Utah Press and was named one of the top 100 books of that year by *Booklist* magazine. He also contributed a piece to the 1995 Henry Holt anthology *Literary Las Vegas*. He has won numerous professional honors, including top awards for writing from the American Association of Sunday and Features Editors, and from the Nevada and California press associations. Although he is a journalist by trade, his fiction has appeared in *The Boston Review, Permafrost,* and *The Chattahoochee Review*. He currently works as an assistant managing editor for the *Reno Gazette-Journal* in Reno, Nevada.

THE MOUNTAINEERS, founded in 1906, is a nonprofit outdoor activity and conservation club, whose mission is "to explore, study, preserve, and enjoy the natural beauty of the outdoors. . . . " Based in Seattle, Washington, the club is now the third-largest such organization in the United States, with 15,000 members and five branches throughout Washington State.

The Mountaineers sponsors both classes and year-round outdoor activities in the Pacific Northwest, which include hiking, mountain climbing, ski-touring, snowshoeing, bicycling, camping, kayaking and canoeing, nature study, sailing, and adventure travel. The club's conservation division supports environmental causes through educational activities, sponsoring legislation, and presenting informational programs. All club activities are led by skilled, experienced volunteers, who are dedicated to promoting safe and responsible enjoyment and preservation of the outdoors.

If you would like to participate in these organized outdoor activities or the club's programs, consider a membership in The Mountaineers. For information and an application, write or call The Mountaineers, Club Headquarters, 300 Third Avenue West, Seattle, Washington 98119; (206) 284-6310.

The Mountaineers Books, an active, nonprofit publishing program of the club, produces guidebooks, instructional texts, historical works, natural history guides, and works on environmental conservation. All books produced by The Mountaineers are aimed at fulfilling the club's mission.

Send or call for our catalog of more than 300 outdoor titles:

The Mountaineers Books
1001 SW Klickitat Way, Suite 201
Seattle, WA 98134
800-553-4453
mbooks@mountaineers.org
www.mountaineersbooks.org